Medical Student Well-Being

Dana Zappetti • Jonathan D. Avery
Editors

Medical Student Well-Being

An Essential Guide

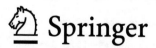 Springer

Editors
Dana Zappetti
Weill Cornell Medical College
New York, NY
USA

Jonathan D. Avery
Cornell University
Weill Cornell Medical College
New York, NY
USA

ISBN 978-3-030-16557-4   ISBN 978-3-030-16558-1   (eBook)
https://doi.org/10.1007/978-3-030-16558-1

This Springer imprint is published by the registered company Springer
Nature Switzerland AG
The registered company address is: Gewerbestrasse 11, 6330 Cham, Switzerland

To current and future students – may you find your way to a wonderful life in medicine

Preface

Medicine finds itself at crossroads. Technology and advances in biomedical science allow us to practice sophisticated medicine using precision techniques and ever-evolving pharmaceuticals to fight disease more successfully than our predecessors. We can cure more, comfort more, and offer more hope to those facing illness. In many ways, it is more satisfying to practice medicine now than ever before. Yet the physician workforce is increasingly burned out and frustrated. Attrition, depression, and suicide are frequent topics of discussion at national meetings, in all specialties of medicine. Why now?

As our profession focuses on the systems issues of medical practice in 2019 – the pros and cons of the electronic medical record, the debate over fee-for-service insurance plans, and how to accomplish the ever-increasing need and interest in access to timely care – our students need to learn skills that will allow them to work within this complicated system and still love the practice of medicine.

It is a privilege to watch students grow from wide-eyed first-year students to seasoned house staff. It is clear that the energy, enthusiasm, and altruism common among our students are the bases for their strength as physicians. We hope that the suggestions and discussions within this book help students to build skills for a successful and happy life in medicine.

New York, NY, USA   Dana Zappetti
New York, NY, USA   Jonathan D. Avery

Contents

List of Contributors

Muhammad Ali, MM, MSS, MA Pastoral Care and Education Department, New York Presbyterian Hospital/Weill Cornell Medical Center, New York, NY, USA

Kerri I. Aronson, MD Pulmonary and Critical Care Medicine, New York Presbyterian Hospital/Weill Cornell Medical College, New York, NY, USA

Jonathan D. Avery, MD Cornell University Weill Cornell Medical College, New York, NY, USA

Joséphine Cool, MD New York Presbyterian Hospital/Weill Cornell Medical College, New York, NY, USA

James M. Dahle, MD, FACEP The White Coat Investor, LLC, Salt Lake City, UT, USA

Stephen Douglas, MDiv, MFA Pastoral Care and Education Department, New York Presbyterian Hospital/Weill Cornell Medical Center, New York, NY, USA

Janna S. Gordon-Elliott, MD New York Presbyterian Hospital/Weill Cornell Medical College, New York, NY, USA

Kristopher A. Kast, MD New York Presbyterian Hospital/Weill Cornell Medical College, New York, NY, USA

Heather Krog, MA Cultural Mentor and Inclusion Facilitator, Copenhagen, Denmark

W. Marcus Lambert, PhD, MS Weill Cornell Medicine, New York, NY, USA

Lisa M. Meeks, PhD, MA University of Michigan Medical School, Department of Family Medicine, Ann Arbor, MI, USA

Joseph F. Murray, MD Weill Cornell Medical College, Department of Psychiatry, New York, NY, USA

Chiti Parikh, MD Weill Cornell Medicine/New York Presbyterian Hospital/Integrative Health and Wellbeing, New York, NY, USA

Paulette Posner, MA Pastoral Care and Education Department, New York Presbyterian Hospital/Weill Cornell Medical Center, New York, NY, USA

Elizabeth Wilson-Anstey, MA, EdD Weill Cornell Medicine, New York, NY, USA

Dana Zappetti, MD Weill Cornell Medical College, New York, NY, USA

Chapter 1
The Physiology of Stress

Joséphine Cool and Dana Zappetti

Allostasis: The Normal Stress Response and the Reason that Stress Exists

All human beings occasionally feel stress. Healthcare workers have jobs that are often demanding physically, mentally, and emotionally and can often be overwhelmed by stress. However, it is important to remember that the stress response exists for a reason. This chapter will review the normal physiologic stress response, examine how this stress response can become dysfunctional and lead to disease, and finally explore the ways that stress can be studied in human beings. This will be framed throughout the chapter with the concepts of allostasis, allostatic load, and allostatic load index.

To start, we will define some terms that will be referred back to throughout this chapter.

J. Cool
New York Presbyterian Hospital/Weill Cornell Medical College, New York, NY, USA
e-mail: joc2059@nyp.org

D. Zappetti (✉)
Weill Cornell Medical College, New York, NY, USA
e-mail: daz9001@med.cornell.edu

Stressor	Any actual or potential disturbance of an individual's environment due to real or perceived noxious stimuli.
Stress mediators	Molecules that bind to receptor targets, act on specific neuronal populations, and have unique downstream effects, for example, catecholamines or cytokines.
Stress response	The activation of coordinated neurophysiological responses in the brain and periphery, through the sympathetic nervous system and the hypothalamic-pituitary-adrenal axis, to respond to the environmental demands caused by stressors. This enables us to adapt to a changing environment.

Stress is difficult to study because its effects on the body are widespread and not easily isolated. Allostasis is a way to conceptualize the reason that our body creates stress. In the original terms, "an organism maintains physiological stability by changing the parameters of its internal milieu by matching them appropriately to environmental demands" [1]. To translate into layman's terms, allostasis indicates achieving stability through change. An example of allostasis in nature would be the accrual of body fat in bears in preparation for hibernation. Allostasis is different from homeostasis in the sense that after the stressor ebbs, there is not necessarily return to the same prestress set point; for example, the bear may not lose all of its hibernation fat when spring arrives.

A normal stress response occurs when the body recognizes a stressor, which can be real or perceived, and thereafter creates a state of heightened vigilance and arousal through the activation of coordinated neurophysiological responses in the brain and in the periphery. A crucial part of the normal stress response is that, after the stressor is removed, there is a recovery phase with return to either the same or a different baseline.

An effective stress response allows us to function in a world with normal development and efficient energy utilization, therefore allowing us to adapt to a changing environment.

We will first illustrate the concept of allostasis with the regulation of heart rate in response to a stressor.

Under normal circumstances, the heart rate is regulated by the autonomic nervous system, i.e., the parasympathetic nervous system (PNS) and the sympathetic nervous system (SNS), which acts on the sinoatrial (SA) node. Prior studies where both propranolol and atropine were administered, so-called double blockade studies, found that the resulting heart rate when the double blockade was present is higher than the normal resting heart rate in the absence of these medications. This implies that vagal dominance, or a basal parasympathetic vagal tone, exists on the SA node that is stronger than the tone exerted by the SNS [2], which allows for energy conservation.

In addition, the PNS has a fast "on and off" effect on the SA node, which leads to a high heart rate variability (HRV) or so-called "beat-to-beat" variability. The reason that the PNS affects the SA node faster than the SNS is secondary to the difference in speed of action of the neurotransmitters characterizing each branch of the ANS. As a reminder, the cardiac parasympathetic pathways start in the nucleus ambiguus of the medulla oblongata (dorsal motor nucleus of the vagus nerve), proceed through the cervical vagus nerves close to the common carotid artery, enter the chest through the mediastinum, and synapse with postganglionic cells on the epicardial surface or within the walls of the heart itself. These cells are close in proximity to the SA and AV nodes. The right vagus nerve predominantly acts on the SA node, and the left vagus nerve predominantly acts on the AV conduction tissue. When the vagus nerve is activated, it leads to release of acetylcholine which acts quickly on muscarinic receptors to decrease the activity of acetylyl cyclase and does not require secondary messengers like cyclic adenosine monophosphate (cAMP), allowing for beat-to-beat control. Indeed, the PNS acts on the order of milliseconds, which allows for the heart to be able to respond quickly to stressors when needed.

In contrast, the cardiac sympathetic pathways start in the intermediolateral columns of the lower cervical and upper thoracic segments of the spinal cord, synapse in the stellate and middle cervical ganglia, then are distributed to the various chambers of the heart via an extensive epicardial plexus and finally penetrate the myocardium along the coronary vessels. The SNS leads to the release of norepinephrine that acts on a beta-adrenergic receptor and leads to an increase in adenylyl cyclase activity. Because the CNS acts through a secondary messenger, its effects are slower. The PNS dominance on the SA node allows for a faster response to a stressor.

To summarize, there is a parasympathetic basal tone that acts on the SA node through the action of the vagus nerve. When a stressor occurs, there are both activation of the SNS and inhibition of the PNS to allow for the heart rate (HR) to increase appropriately. The SNS and PNS are themselves under control of a central autonomic network located in the brain.

When a stressor occurs, for example, a decrease in blood pressure from blood loss, baroreceptors in the aortic arch and carotid sinuses send afferent signals to the central autonomic network in the brain. This leads to inhibition of the vagus nerve through GABAergic neurons and release of the PNS basal tone on the SA node and allows for an increase in heart rate and therefore cardiac output [2].

The central autonomic network is itself under regulation of several areas in the brain, which means that at the highest level the brain is the gatekeeper of the stress response. In a very simplified manner, just like there is tonic inhibition of the SA node by the PNS, in the brain, there is tonic inhibition of the amygdala by the prefrontal cortex [2]. Other brain regions included in this process are the premotor cortex, frontal lobe, hypothalamus, temporal lobe, and cingulate gyrus. The amygdala is continuously assessing the threats and regulates the perception of fear, but the prefrontal cortex tonically inhibits this to prevent the presence of a continuous

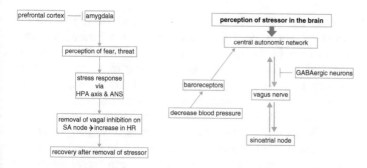

FIGURE 1.1 The autonomic system regulates the stress response

stress response. Perception of a stressor leads to release of this tonic inhibition, which allows for activation of the stress response via the HPA axis and the ANS. As discussed above, this leads to removal of vagal inhibition on the SA node and therefore an increase in the HR. To bring this back to the concepts introduced earlier, in this scenario, *allostasis* means that there is an increase in the heart rate in response to a stressor, but also recovery of the HR after removal of the stressor (Fig. 1.1).

The Hypothalamic-Pituitary-Adrenal Axis

As mentioned earlier, the purpose of a normal stress response is to summon additional energy in response to stress. The brain and the central autonomic network ultimately regulate when the stress response is activated, usually in response to visceral and sensory stimuli that reach the brain through ascending brainstem pathways and limbic pathways. Once it is activated, the stress response proceeds via the HPA axis, which is a neuroendocrine system that is the major stress system in the body, leading to the production of cortisol by the adrenal gland.

In more detail, when the brain agrees that the body needs to respond to a stressor, the parvocellular neurons of the *hypothalamic* paraventricular nucleus (PVN) are activated, which leads to the release of *corticotropin-releasing hormone* (CRH) and vasopressin. These hormones in turn act in the *anterior pituitary* via CRHR1 to process pro-opiomelanocortin (POMC) to *corticotropin* (ACTH), opioid, and melanocortin peptides. ACTH then acts on the *adrenal cortex* to secrete *cortisol* in humans. As a reminder, the adrenal gland is composed of the medulla and the cortex. The medulla secretes catecholamines (epinephrine and norepinephrine); the cortex is divided into three zones: the outermost zona glomerulosa, which secretes aldosterone; the middle zone fasciculata, which secretes glucocorticoids; and the zona reticularis, which secretes androgens such as dehydroepiandrosterone (DHEA).

Cortisol is a glucocorticoid that affects numerous tissues to mobilize or store energy [3]. It alters glucose and fat metabolism, bone metabolism, cardiovascular responsiveness, and the immune system. Cortisol mediates the stress response in a biphasic manner through immediate and delayed responses.

The Fast and Slow Paths of the Stress Response

The *fast effect* of cortisol, which acts within milliseconds, is characterized by the release of catecholamines and neuropeptides such as norepinephrine, serotonin, dopamine, and CRH that lead to increased vigilance, alertness, arousal, and attention. The mechanism of the rapid responses is poorly understood but is thought to involve the binding of cortisol to the mineralocorticoid receptor (MR) in the brain leading to conformational changes and reaggregation with other proteins such as heat-shock proteins [3].

The *slow effect* of cortisol starts within 1–2 hours after stressor exposure. It is initiated when cortisol binds to both MRs and glucocorticoid receptors (GRs) in the brain, which leads to changes in gene transcription and therefore expression of proteins that affect neuronal function. This allows for the reorganization of resources to mobilize them on a longer time scale. Changes in cell metabolism, structure, and synaptic transmission are mediated by the altered expression of 70–100 genes through the activation of MRs or GRs in the hippocampus.

However, MRs and GRs have different cellular and behavioral effects. MRs, which in the brain lack specificity for aldosterone, are implicated in the appraisal process and are mainly involved in the fast effect at the onset of the stress response. MRs are located in the hippocampus, the amygdala paraventricular nucleus (PVN), and the locus coeruleus and therefore help with the cognitive, emotional, and neuroendocrine processing of stressful events. GRs have a tenfold higher threshold of activation than MRs and are ubiquitous in the brain but mainly located in the hippocampus and parvocellular nucleus. They are more involved in the slow effect of the stress response via changes in gene transcription and are also essential in the termination of the stress response via negative feedback regulation. GRs also help prepare for future stressors by promoting memory storage. Research in rats [4, 5] has shown that early adverse life events or chronic stress in adulthood led to a decrease in the number of functioning GRs in the hippocampus, presumably leading to deficient memory storage of stressors and termination of the stress response.

Although MRs and GRs seem to mediate many of the effects of the stress response, further research [6] has also shown that there may be other membrane-associated receptors such as G-protein-coupled receptors that are also involved.

Changes in Stressor Type Can Lead to Changes in Mediator

Different types of stress can activate varied areas of the brain. For example, physical stressors such as blood loss, trauma, or cold lead to preferential activation of the brainstem and hypothalamic regions. Psychological stressors such as social embarrassment or deadlines lead to preferential activation of the amygdala and prefrontal cortex (for emotion and decision-making) and hippocampus (for memory). Similarly, the duration of a stressor can affect which mediator is used in the stress response. Stress mediators include but are not limited to catecholamines, dopamine, serotonin, CRH, urocortins, vasopressin, orexin, dynorphin, corticosteroids, neurosteroids, insulin, ghrelin, and leptin. These different mediators act preferentially on different areas of the brain and can lead to varied end effects. For example, norepinephrine can act on the locus coeruleus to shift the processing of information from focused to general scanning; dopamine released from the prefrontal cortex allows for better risk assessment; and CRH of course leads to the activation of ACTH in the anterior pituitary but is also released in the amygdala, hippocampus, and locus coeruleus to enhance memory consolidation [4].

Allostatic Load: When the Stress Response Becomes Pathological

As described above, allostasis is a way to conceptualize the normal physiologic stress response that includes a period of activity followed by a period of recovery.

Allostatic load describes the wear and tear of the body from stress and inefficient allostasis [7]. This wear and tear can include genetic load, life experiences such as major life events or trauma, and health habits and determines the resilience to stress. In contrast to allostasis, in allostatic load, there is no normal return to baseline after removal of the stressor. Based on the model set in place by McEwen, there are four main ways in which allostatic states deviate from healthy responses. The first is in the setting of repeated hits. If one gets repeated hits of the same stressor in short periods of time, there is not enough time to habituate to the recurrence of the same stressor. The second manner, which is an extension of the first, is through lack of adaptation. Not only is one unable to habituate to repeated stressors, but with each hit, one is less efficient and less capable of responding appropriately to the stressor. The third way in which allostatic load can develop is when there is a prolonged response to a stressor without recovery after the stressor is removed. And finally, the fourth way in which allostatic load can occur is through the development of an inadequate response, i.e., that the normal physiologic stress response is not elicited at all (Fig. 1.2).

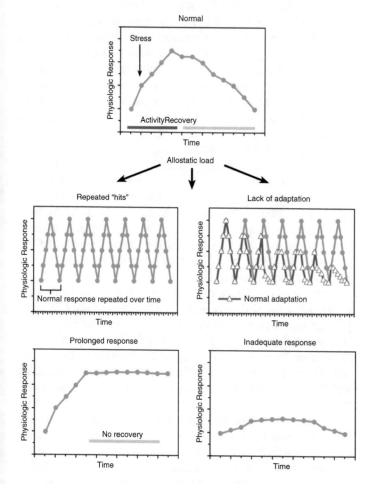

FIGURE. 1.2 Development of allostatic load [7]

Allostatic load therefore means that there is either an inadequate stress response or an inadequate recovery to the stress response.

When a stressor occurs, *primary mediators*, such as stress hormones and their antagonists, pro- and anti-inflammatory cytokines (IL6, TNF-alpha), etc., exert *primary effects* on cellular processes by changing the activity of enzymes, receptors, ion channels, and genes. In a normal allostatic response, these primary effects ebb once the stress response ends. However, when these primary effects are allowed to proceed unfettered without recovery, they lead to *secondary outcomes*, or detrimental changes in metabolic, cardiovascular, and immune functions to subclinical levels. This can include increase in insulin resistance, cholesterol, blood pressure, CRP, etc. When the stress response proceeds even further, these secondary outcomes lead to *tertiary outcomes*, i.e., disease and death, indicating *allostatic overload*.

Bringing this back to the example of tachycardia described previously, if there is no brake on the brain's perception of fear and threat, then the stress response can proceed unfettered via the HPA axis and the ANS. This leads to continuous removal of vagal inhibition on the SA node, constantly elevated heart rate, and no recovery after removal of the stressor. Therefore, even after the stressor is removed, the heart rate stays elevated [2].

Decreased heart rate variability can lead to an increase in inflammation and deregulation of glucose and the HPA axis [2]. Furthermore, from twin studies, it seems that a low HRV is also a risk factor for depression [8], all examples of allostatic load. Beyond just looking at the heart rate, autonomic imbalance in general is thought to be involved in both acute and chronic stresses and is associated with heart disease, diabetes, and obesity [9].

In life, factors that can lead to continued stress and allostatic load can be thought of as coming from multiple levels, as described by McEwen [7]. First, the macro-system includes stressors linked to socioeconomic status such as education and income, ethnicity, and spirituality. Second, the exo-system includes stressors from neighborhood location such as crowd-ing, noise, lack of housing, and social networks. Third, the micro-system includes stressors from family, work, and peer groups. Finally, stressors can come from the individual includ-ing from personality and genetics.

Allostatic Load in the Brain

Studying the effects of stress on the brain has been mainly done in rats, or in post-mortem studies in humans. Areas of the brain that are involved in the stress response, such as the hippocampus, the prefrontal cortex, and the amygdala, often grouped together as the limbic system, can undergo structural change in the presence of both acute and chronic stresses [7]. For example, glucocorticoids can affect structural plastic-ity by increasing neurogenesis during physical activity [10]. Conversely, rats that have been maternally deprived have a decrease in adult-generated immature neurons and impaired negative feedback to the HPA axis [11]. Prolonged emo-tional stressors can also lead to long-term alterations in the limbic system [12]; for instance, patients that suffered from prolonged mood disorders often had a decrease in density and/or expression of corticosteroid receptors in the limbic forebrain [12, 13]. To compound the problem, damage to the hippocampus can lead to a more prolonged stress response, creating a vicious cycle.

The Allostatic Load Index Groups Allostatic Load Biomarkers and Is a Way to Study Allostatic Load, or Stress, in Medicine

The impact of stress on the human body is difficult to study because its effects are so widespread and affect many differ-ent organ systems simultaneously. The allostatic load index is one way to make the pathological effects of stress measurable and discuss it in a consistent way. It groups various biomarkers that mirror the secondary outcomes discussed above into an index. These biomarkers are diverse and stem from the cardiovascular and respiratory system (such as systolic blood pressure and HRV), metabolic system (such as LDL, triglycerides, GFR, and insulin), neuroendocrine system (such as DHEA-S and cortisol levels), anthropometric system (such as height, BMI, and % fat), and immune system (such as ESR and CRP). The first study to include an allostatic load index [14] used 12-hour urinary cortisol, epinephrine, and norepinephrine output, serum DHEA-S, total cholesterol-to-HDL ratio, HDL, A1c, aggregate systolic and diastolic blood pressure, and waist-to-hip ratio. They found that higher allostatic load was associated with lower baseline functioning, poorer cognitive performance, and weaker physical performance. One recent meta-analysis [15] performed a meta-analysis of allostatic load studies and showed that the most frequently used biomarkers are metabolic, neuroendocrine, and cardiovascular; immune biomarkers are less frequently used but are very quickly increasing in frequency. Further studies have found that regardless of age, decreases in allostatic load are associated with reductions in risk of dying earlier [16].

The allostatic load index can also be used to examine the relationship between socioeconomic stressors and poor outcomes later in life. For instance, a cohort study over 6 years [17] found that poverty led to more significant increase in allostatic load until middle age and that older poorer individuals with high allostatic load had a life expectancy that was 6 years shorter than those with low biological risk, compared to individuals matched for income and sex. Similarly, data from NHANES [18] showed that allostatic load was found to soften the effects of education and income gradients in the prediction of ischemic heart disease.

Another recent study [19] used the allostatic load index to examine whether adverse childhood experiences (ACEs), measured prospectively with data collected at ages 7, 11, and 16 via the National Child Development Study in the UK, affected health in middle age. They calculated an allostatic load index based on data from a biomedical survey collected at age 44; their index encompassed 14 parameters including salivary cortisol t1 (nanomoles per liter), salivary cortisol t1–t2 (nanomoles per liter), insulin-like growth factor-1 (IGF1), CRP, fibrinogen, IgE, HDL, LDL, TG, A1c, SBP, DBP, HR, and peak expiratory flow. They found that factors associated with a significantly higher allostatic load in men included father's social class at birth, mother's overweight BMI at birth, low birth weight, and smoking at age 23.

The allostatic load index can be compared to the intelligence quotient (IQ), which allows us to measure intelligence, something that we also do not understand completely. The largest downside of the allostatic load index is that there is not yet a consensus as to what biomarkers it should consistently include, which makes studies using the allostatic load index difficult to compare. This is partly because we are continuing to learn more about how stress affects the body physiologically and thereby revisiting the importance of known biomarkers, or discovering new biomarkers that can be included, such as various cytokines or rheumatological markers.

As physicians and scientists, we feel stress in life and career. Understanding that our response to this stress is biological and important in our ability to overcome the stressor is imperative. Some amount of stress is good—it allows us to study for that important exam, remain awake to complete a research proposal, and can increase our focus. Allowing the stress response to be sustained, however, can be debilitating to our central nervous system, mind, and body.

References

1. Sterling P, Allostasis EJ. A new paradigm to explain arousal pathology. In: Handbook of life stress, cognition and health. New York: Wiley; 1988. p. 629–49.
2. Thayer JF, Ahs F, Fredrikson M, Sollers JJ, Wager TD. A meta-analysis of heart rate variability and neuroimaging studies: implications for heart rate variability as a marker of stress and health. Neurosci Biobehav Rev. 2012;36(2):747–56. https://doi.org/10.1016/j.neubiorev.2011.11.009.

3. De Kloet ER, Joëls M, Holsboer F. Stress and the brain: from adaptation to disease. Nat Rev Neurosci. 2005;6(6):463–75. https://doi.org/10.1038/nrn1683.

4. Joëls M, Baram TZ. The neuro-symphony of stress. Nat Rev Neurosci. 2009;10(6):459–66. https://doi.org/10.1038/nrn2632.

5. Champagne DL, et al. Maternal care and hippocampal plasticity: evidence for experience-dependent structural plasticity, altered synaptic functioning, and differential responsiveness to glucocorticoids and stress. J Neurosci. 2008;28(23):6037–45.

6. McEwen BS, Nasca C, Gray JD. Stress effects on neuronal structure: hippocampus, amygdala, and prefrontal cortex. Neuropsychopharmacology. 2016;41(1):3.

7. McEwen BS. Physiology and neurobiology of stress and adaptation: central role of the brain. Physiol Rev. 2007;87(3):873–904. https://doi.org/10.1152/physrev.00041.2006.

8. Huang M, et al. Association of depressive symptoms and heart rate variability in Vietnam war–era twins: a longitudinal twin difference study. JAMA Psychiat. 2018;75(7):705–12.

9. Wulsin L, Herman J, Thayer JF. Stress, autonomic imbalance, and the prediction of metabolic risk: a model and a proposal for research. Neurosci Biobehav Rev. 2017;86:12–20.

10. Mirescu C, Gould E. Stress and adult neurogenesis. Hippocampus. 2006;16(3):233–8. Web

11. Mirescu C, Peters JD, Gould E. Early life experience alters response of adult neurogenesis to stress. Nat Neurosci. 2004;7(8):841.

12. Radley J, et al. Chronic stress and brain plasticity: mechanisms underlying adaptive and maladaptive changes and implications for stress-related CNS disorders. Neurosci Biobehav Rev. 2015;58:79–91.

13. Alt SR, et al. Differential expression of glucocorticoid receptor transcripts in major depressive disorder is not epigenetically programmed. Psychoneuroendocrinology. 2010;35(4):544–56.

14. Seeman TE, et al. Price of adaptation—allostatic load and its health consequences: MacArthur studies of successful aging. Arch Intern Med. 1997;157(19):2259–68.

15. Juster R-P, McEwen BS, Lupien SJ. Allostatic load biomarkers of chronic stress and impact on health and cognition. Neurosci Biobehav Rev. 2010;35(1):2–16. https://doi.org/10.1016/j.neubiorev.2009.10.002.

16. Karlamangla AS, Singer BH, Seeman TE. Reduction in allostatic load in older adults is associated with lower all-cause mortality risk: MacArthur studies of successful aging. Psychosom Med. 2006;68(3):500–7.

17. Crimmins EM, Kim JK, Seeman TE. Poverty and biological risk: the earlier "aging" of the poor. J Gerontol A Biol Sci Med Sci. 2009;64(2):286–92. https://doi.org/10.1093/gerona/gln010.

18. Sabbah W, Watt RG, Sheiham A, Tsakos G. Effects of allostatic load on the social gradient in ischaemic heart disease and periodontal disease: evidence from the Third National Health and Nutrition Examination Survey. J Epidemiol Community Health. 2008;62(5):415–20. https://doi.org/10.1136/jech.2007.064188.

19. Barboza Solís C, Kelly-Irving M, Fantin R, et al. Adverse childhood experiences and physiological wear-and-tear in midlife: findings from the 1958 British birth cohort. Proc Natl Acad Sci U S A. 2015;112(7):E738–46. https://doi.org/10.1073/pnas.1417325112.

Chapter 2
Mental Health and Medical Education

Lisa M. Meeks and Joseph F. Murray

Introduction

Medicine attracts candidates who are highly driven, competitive, compassionate, intelligent, and goal oriented. They have already succeeded at getting into a medical school, a challenging task. And yet, we know that medical students experience anxiety and depressive symptoms at greater rates than the general population [6]. Over 25% of medical students have experienced major depression symptoms, and more than 10% of students have experienced suicidal ideation [30]. How is it that high-achieving students who have succeeded at matriculating into medical school struggle so much?

One model that attempts to explain how and why mental health disorders are expressed in some individuals and not others is the diathesis-stress model [25]. This model suggests that mental health disorders may be the result of an interac-

L. M. Meeks (✉)
University of Michigan Medical School, Department of Family Medicine, Ann Arbor, MI, USA
e-mail: meeksli@med.umich.edu

J. F. Murray
Weill Cornell Medical College, Department of Psychiatry, New York, NY, USA
e-mail: jfmurray@med.cornell.edu

© Springer Nature Switzerland AG 2019
D. Zappetti, J. D. Avery (eds.), *Medical Student Well-Being*,
https://doi.org/10.1007/978-3-030-16558-1_2

tion between a pre-disposed vulnerability to a mental health condition (e.g., genetic makeup, family history, early losses or traumas, personality characteristics, social supports) and a stressor caused by life experiences. In addition, there are certain mental health disorders that are present in late adolescents, the same time that traditional students are entering medical school. Thus, is it possible that the unique stressors of medical school—and the age of the average medical student— may result in a worsening of mental health and well-being?

In this chapter, we aim to:

1. Identify some of the more common mental health disorders that occur in the medical student population (the young adult demographic).
2. Examine the climate of medicine, medical education, and accompanying LCME guidance for wellness.
3. Explore factors that can impact medical students' overall well-being and mental health.
4. Introduce key concepts of disability accommodations and insurance.
5. Review key take-home points.

Overview of Mental Health Disorders

Medical students can experience a wide range of mental health challenges. For some, maintaining mental health may be a lifelong struggle, one that is mitigated by supports (e.g., therapy, medication, social networks, exercise, and good sleep hygiene). For others, mental health challenges may be new and may be falsely dismissed as part of the normative transition to medical school. Medical students are not immune to the wide range of mental health issues that can be seen in the young adult demographic, including but not limited to anxiety disorders, mood disorders, eating disorders, substance use disorders, trauma and stressor-related disorders, obsessive-compulsive disorders, psychotic disorders, personality disorders, and sleep disorders. This chapter will focus on some of the more common anxiety disorders and mood disorders, as these can affect a wide range of medical students and have been well studied. Unless otherwise noted, the descriptions of the symptoms and the demographic information related to the specific anxiety and mood disorders in this chapter are taken from the DSM V (2013).

Anxiety Disorders

Anxiety disorders are the most common psychiatric (mental health) disorders, especially in childhood and adolescence, where most typically have their onset. Given the demographic profile of medical students (most are in their 20s or 30s), a subset of students will have had an anxiety disorder earlier in their lives, be currently diagnosed with an anxiety disorder, or may struggle with anxiety that is partially treated. According to the National Institute of Mental Health, an estimated 22.3% of adults ages 18–29 and 22.7% of adults ages 30–44 had an anxiety disorder in 2016 [28].

Anxiety disorders generally involve a heightened fear response beyond what one would normally expect, tension and vigilance in preparation for future danger, and cautious or avoidant behaviors. The heightened fear response might culminate in a panic attack, where the person experiences an abrupt surge of intense fear or discomfort that could include symptoms like heart racing, sweating, trembling, shortness of breath, choking, chest discomfort/pain, nausea, abdominal distress, dizziness, lightheadedness, chills, heat, numbness, or tingling. During a panic attack, a person might feel that he/she is going crazy or worries that he/she will die. He/she might also feel like he/she is having an out-of-body experience or that his/her symptoms are not real.

Some of the most common anxiety disorders we see in the medical school population include:

1. *Specific phobia* is a marked fear about an object or situation, out of proportion to the situation or context. This fear causes distress and impairs one's functioning. The person might avoid the feared situation or object, or he/she might

try to endure it with great difficulty. Some examples include fear of flying, heights, animals, bridges, tunnels, receiving an injection, seeing blood, etc. The onset is typically in childhood, sometimes after a traumatic experience. Rates of the disorder peak in adolescence. The prevalence estimate is 7–9%, and women tend to outnumber men.

Impact on Medical Students Some students with phobias of bridges, tunnels, or flying might have challenges in *getting to* certain clinical rotations. Medical students travel to different cities or states during the residency application process as well. Some students with blood or injection phobias may have difficulty *during* clinical rotations. In these cases, the phobia could limit the student's educational experiences and career opportunities or even their ability to persist and graduate.

> **Tip**
> Students should seek treatment during the first year of medical school for specific phobias. These phobias can limit their opportunities and they are treatable.

2. *Social anxiety disorder* (social phobia) is a marked fear about social situations where the individual is exposed to possible scrutiny by others. This could happen in social interactions, meeting people, having a conversation, being observed, or performing in front of others (like presenting a patient during rounds). The person worries that he/she will show anxiety symptoms or act in a way that will be viewed negatively (e.g., will be humiliating, embarrassing, or lead to rejection). The fear is out of proportion to the context and causes distress or impairment in functioning. Sometimes the anxiety is limited to performance and not present in other social situations. The age of onset for 75% of people with the disorder is between 8 and 15 years. Adulthood onset is less common, and it may follow a stress-

ful or humiliating experience or life changes with new social roles. The prevalence estimate is 7%, and women outnumber men.

Impact on Medical Students   Starting medical school, students come into a new environment where they know few people. The process of meeting and getting to know many people while making a major life change is stressful for anyone, but it can be particularly challenging for someone with social anxiety disorder. This might limit the student's ability to create a social support network. In the classroom and on clinical rotation, much of the teaching, learning, and evaluation might occur in small group settings where discussion is required and evaluated. Eventually students will be called upon to present patients and may be subject to rapid-fire questioning about medical knowledge in front of the team, which can be particularly difficult for students with social anxiety disorder. Some students with social anxiety disorder might also experience major depression and substance use disorders as a result of trying to mitigate their anxiety with substance use.

Tip
Students who experience anxiety while engaging in small group discussions or presentations should reach out to counseling for assistance. Performance can improve, and students will enjoy the experience.

Tip
Students who experience anxiety about presenting patients or clinical encounters with patients may find relief using the basic principles of systematic desensitization, whereby schools expose the student to incremental patient encounters or patient presentations using a simulation lab and standardized patients.

3. *Panic disorder* consists of recurrent, unexpected panic attacks that result in excessive worry about future attacks, the consequences of an attack, or a significant change in behavior related to the attacks. Onset can occur in childhood but more commonly in adolescence or adulthood. Prevalence is estimated to be 2–3%, with women outnumbering men 2:1.

Some people with panic disorder also have *agoraphobia*.

Agoraphobia is a marked fear about situations where escape might be difficult or where help might not be available in the event of a panic attack or other symptoms. This must occur in two or more of the following situations: public transportation, open spaces, enclosed spaces, standing in line/being in a crowd, or being outside of the home alone. Onset can occur in adolescence or adulthood. The mean age of onset is 17 years old. The prevalence is 1.7%, and women outnumber men.

Impact on Medical Students Students with panic disorder and/or agoraphobia can engage in avoidance behaviors, e.g., missing class, skipping large groups, making early exits, and engaging in fewer social opportunities. This avoidance can negatively impact their academic performance as well as their overall social well-being. Some students with panic disorder and/or agoraphobia might also experience major depression.

Tip
Students who experience panic attacks while on the wards can use bathroom stalls as safe space to regroup and meditate or medicate. Bathrooms are usually close by when students feel an impending attack, and social graces dictate that others do not place critical inquiry on time spent in a restroom, giving the student a short but much needed and socially accepted reprieve.

4. *Generalized anxiety disorder* consists of excessive anxiety and worry (apprehensive expectation) about several events or activities. The worry is hard to control and is associated with heightened anxiety symptoms, and it causes distress or impairment in one's functioning. Half of all people who develop the disorder do so before the age of 30. Onset can begin in adolescence. The prevalence is 2.9%, and women outnumber men.

Impact on Medical Students The student with generalized anxiety disorder often worries about things that we might view as minor and require a great deal of reassurance. Difficulty with sleep is a common symptom of generalized anxiety disorder, and the student might show up late in the morning or appear tired. As a result, the student with generalized anxiety disorder might also experience major depression. It is important to remember that anxiety is a downward spiral that can quickly become worrisome. Small changes in behavior, that at first appear normative to the transition to medical school, may actually be the beginning of an anxiety disorder (see Fig. 2.1).

Anxiety Symptoms in Medical School While it is difficult to measure how many medical students experience anxiety disorders, some attempts have been made to look at anxiety symptoms in general. (Indeed, many of those symptoms are those of generalized anxiety disorder.) In a systematic review of depression, anxiety, and other indicators of psychological distress among US and Canadian medical students, the authors noted that several studies showed higher rates of anxiety symptoms among medical students compared to the general population [6].

Treatment of Anxiety Disorders The standard treatments for anxiety disorders include psychotherapy and/or pharmacotherapy. Cognitive-behavioral therapy (CBT) is one of the most frequently used treatment modalities, and it can be

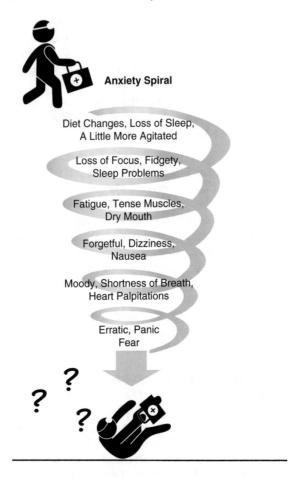

FIGURE 2.1 Anxiety spiral (Illustrated by: Amy Rutherford 2019)

used for all anxiety disorders. In addition, psychodynamic psychotherapy can be used for panic disorder. Psychiatric medication can be helpful in lessening the anxiety symptoms. Antidepressants like the selective serotonin reuptake inhibitors (SSRIs) or antianxiety agents like buspirone are daily medications used in the treatment of anxiety disorders. Other medications are fast acting and can be taken only as needed, like beta-blockers for performance or social anxiety disorder and benzodiazepines for anxiety associated with panic or panic attacks. For those with panic or performance anxieties, sometimes just having the medication nearby lessens the anxiety.

Mood Disorders

The most common mood disorders are major depressive disorder and bipolar disorder.

1. *Major depressive disorder* (sometimes commonly called "depression") is characterized by a major depressive episode: at least 2 weeks of persistently low mood or loss of ability to enjoy things, accompanied by several other symptoms, including changes in weight/appetite or sleep, impaired concentration, fatigue/low energy, agitation or retardation, worthlessness, excessive or inappropriate guilt, or recurrent thoughts of death or suicidal thoughts, plan, or attempt. These symptoms cause impairment in the person's functioning. Some episodes can be severe, causing significant impairment. The consequences can also be worrisome, including an increased risk of suicide.

The incidence of major depressive disorder begins to climb at puberty, reaching a peak in the 20s. Women tend to have 1.5- to 3-fold higher rates than men beginning in early adolescence. According to the National Institute of Mental Health (NIMH), the past year prevalence of a major depressive episode among adults nationwide in 2016 was 10.9% (ages 18–25) and 7.4% (ages 26–49) [28].

In a systematic review and meta-analysis of the prevalence of depression, depressive symptoms, and suicidal ideation among medical students, Rotenstein et al. [30] found that overall prevalence of depression or depressive symptoms in medical students was 27.2%. In studies that assessed depressive symptoms before and during medical school, the median absolute increase in symptoms during medical school was

13.5%. The various indices used in the studies showed depressive symptom prevalence to be 2.2 to 5.2 times higher among medical students than individuals of similar age in the general population. The percentage of students screening positive for depression who sought psychiatric treatment was 15.7%. The overall prevalence of suicidal ideation was 11.1% [30].

Impact on Medical Students The medical student with major depressive disorder often struggle silently. Some depressive symptoms, like trouble with sleep, concentration, appetite, and energy, can impair the student's ability to function at a high level. They often curtail social activities due to fatigue and loss of enjoyment, impairing their social engagement and ability to create a social support network. Medical students are at greater risk of suicidal thoughts and potentially suicide attempts. The data from Rotenstein et al. [30] showing that over one quarter of medical students experienced symptoms of major depression and that, of those who experience those symptoms, only 15.7% received treatment is worrisome. There is a tremendous amount of silent suffering among medical students, who may view the symptoms of depression and anxiety as part of the norm in the profession of medicine.

> **Tip**
> Students who lose the ability to enjoy things that usually bring them pleasure may be experiencing anhedonia, one of the key symptoms of major depression.

Treatment of Major Depressive Disorder Psychotherapy can be an effective treatment for mild and possibly moderate episodes of depression. CBT is the most commonly used modality, and IPT (interpersonal therapy) has been shown to be beneficial. Antidepressant medication can be used alone or in conjunction with psychotherapy, and it is necessary for moderate to severe episodes of the disorder, while hospitalization is sometimes required for severe episodes. There are other non-medication treatments including ECT (electroconvulsive therapy) and TMS (transcranial magnetic stimulation). Novel treatments for major depressive disorder include the use of the dissociative anesthetic ketamine.

2. *Bipolar disorder* is a mood disorder where individuals experience episodes that can include increased energy, decreased need for sleep, inflated self-esteem or grandiosity, more talkative or pressured speech, racing thoughts or flight of ideas, distractibility, increase in goal-directed activity, and excessive involvement in risky activities. Depending on the degree and duration, these episodes can be called manic or hypomanic. Many individuals also experience depressive episodes, and some experience mixed episodes (symptoms with both mania and depression).

The prevalence of bipolar 1 disorder (with the presence of at least one manic episode) is 0.6%, and age of onset is late teens to early 20s. The prevalence of bipolar 2 disorder (with the presence of at least one hypomanic episode and at least one depressive episode) is 0.8%, and the average of onset is the mid-20s. Men may slightly outnumber women, although some data show similar prevalence rates. The suicide risk in bipolar disorder is high. Estimates are that up to a third of those with bipolar disorder may attempt suicide, up to 15 times that of the general population.

Impact on Medical Students The student with bipolar disorder in a manic or hypomanic episode might present with behavioral disruption and hard-to-follow thinking and demonstrate poor impulse control. Often a student needs to be on a short leave to treat the episode and make adjustments to medication. Sometimes this requires psychiatric hospitalization.

Treatment of Bipolar Disorder The mainstay of treatment for bipolar disorder is pharmacotherapy with mood-stabilizing medications. There are some psychotherapies that can also be helpful in the management of bipolar disorder. For some episodes of mania, hypomania, or depression in bipolar disorder, hospitalization can not only be beneficial but also sometimes necessary.

> **Tip**
> Medical students with a history of mental health concerns or treatment should get connected to a mental health provider as soon as they arrive at school. Establishing care and a relationship with a provider is imperative, even when things are going well.

The Environment: Are We at Crisis Level?

In a recent commentary, leaders from the National Academy of Medicine, the Association of American Medical Colleges, and the Accreditation Council for Graduate Medical Education declared that clinician burnout, depression, and suicide had reached a "crisis level" [11, 27].

As a community, we continue to examine the impact of medical education on our students and examine the underlying causes. Recognizing the unique structure of medical education (e.g., the volume of information, inherent stressors in caring for others, long hours, difficult patients, poor learning environments, financial concerns, information overload, and career planning), it is easy to understand that medical education will likely represent the most stressful time in the student's life to date.

Burnout

Burnout is just one sign that medicine and mental health do not always align. We know that burnout, most often defined as a function of three indicators, emotional exhaustion associated with work-related stress, feelings of detachment toward patients, and a low sense of personal accomplishment, is higher among physicians than in many other fields [33, 34]. Medical students, however, are not immune to this phenomenon, with more than half of medical students reporting symptoms of burnout [9, 10]. Physicians often experience burnout as a result of lack of control over schedule, time pressures, and the chaotic work environment inherent in medicine [20]. These environmental contributors hold true for medical students and are exacerbated by the transition to medical school, lack of sleep, volume of information, lack of time to engage in social supports, and the first-time exposure to suffering and death.

Burnout is a precursor to other unhealthy behaviors in medical students including unprofessional behavior [8], substance abuse [15], dropping out of medical school [9], and suicide [7]. Remember that the effects of burnout impact over 50% of medical students and can be accompanied by devastating consequences (see Fig. 2.2).

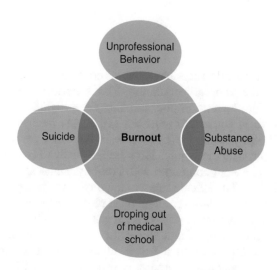

FIGURE 2.2 The impact of burnout on medical students

Depression

The data on the presence of depressive symptoms and depression among medical students paints a worrisome picture. In a study assessing levels of stress and depressive symptoms in two classes of students at one medical school, the number of students found to be at risk for depression in their first year of medical school was 28.4% in the second year and 39% in the third year [21].

A systematic review and meta-analysis of the depression and suicidal ideation among medical students noted an overall prevalence of depressive symptoms or depression in medical students was 27.2%. In those studies that compared depressive symptoms before and during medical school, the mean absolute increase in symptoms during medical school was 13.5%. The presence of suicidal ideation is also of concern, for among medical students, 11.1% reported having thoughts of suicide. Of those students who screened positive for depression, the percentage who sought psychiatric treatment was only 15.7% [30].

Suicide

Physician suicide rates have been known to be higher than that of the general population. The American Foundation for Suicide Prevention put out a fact sheet highlighting some of the most important statistics [1]. It has been estimated that 300 physicians die by suicide in the USA per year [5]. Physicians who died by suicide were less likely to be in mental health treatment compared with non-physicians who died by suicide [13]. The suicide rate among physicians is higher than the general population: among male physicians, it is 1.41 times higher; among female physicians, it is 2.27 times higher [31].

A recent study about the causes of death of residents in Accreditation Council for Graduate Medical Education (ACGME)-accredited programs from 2000 to 2014 noted that suicide was the fourth leading cause of death among female residents, but the leading cause of death among male residents. A majority of the suicides occurred in the first 2 years of training. The overall death rate by suicide was lower among the residents compared to the population at large, although when the residents were broken into age groups, both men and women residents in the 35–44 and the 45–54 years age groups had a higher suicide rates than the general population [37].

With data showing the presence of suicidal ideation among medical students at 11.1%, what are the actual rates of medical student suicides [30]? This question is difficult to answer. Some earlier, limited studies showed suicide rates lower than the general population. With no central database and no organized way of connecting the cause of death (suicide) with occupation (student vs. medical student), it is hard to generate reliable data. Additionally, if a student dies, families have no obligation to communicate with the cause of death [4]. There is a need for a better way of measuring suicides among medical students in order to formulate better preventative measures.

Tip
Students having thoughts of suicide should have access to an emergency contact person at the school, and the National Suicide Prevention Hotline should be posted in multiple, easy-to-access locations (online, student handbook, badge stickers). The NSPH number is 1–800–273-8255 and is staffed 24/7.

Lack of Help-Seeking Behavior in Medical Education

Medical students are perceptive. They pick up on the stigma of depression and mental illness and worry that having a mental health challenge will harm their chances of honoring, matching, and securing licensure. Even if students sought treatment prior to medical school, they might not seek treatment in medical school. In a 2002 study, researchers found that medical students are reluctant to disclose in this new setting over concerns about a lack of confidentiality, stigma associated with using mental health services, cost, fear of documentation on academic record, and fear of unwanted intervention [12]. More recent studies confirm this fear of stigma among medical students with identified psychological disabilities [24].

Liaison Committee on Medical Education (LCME) Guidelines for Medical Student Health Services

In response to the growing need for mental health services for medical students, the Liaison Committee on Medical Education (LCME), the accrediting body for schools leading to the M.D. degree in the USA, added three elements that must be followed in order to maintain accreditation (see Table 2.1) [19]. These elements necessitate that counseling services are in place to promote well-being and facilitate adjustment to medical school (12.3); that students have timely access to needed diagnostic, preventive, and therapeutic health services in reasonable proximity to the locations of clinical rotations; that students are excused to seek needed care (12.4); and that providers of mental health services have no involvement in the academic assessment or promotion of the medical students and maintained records in accordance with legal requirements for security, privacy, confidentiality, and accessibility (12.5). The LCME's guidance to medical schools helps schools understand their responsibility for supporting medical student well-being.

Many of the services offered in medical school are in *response* to poor mental health, versus an attempt to *proactively mitigate* mental health distress and build resilience. To proactively address mental health and wellness, school officials must first understand the specific factors contributing to the decline in medical student well-being.

TABLE 2.1 LCME requirements for health-care services and well-being programs

12.3 Personal Counseling/Well-Being Programs A medical school has in place an effective system of personal counseling for its medical students that includes programs to promote their well-being and to facilitate their adjustment to the physical and emotional demands of medical education.
12.4 Student Access to Health-Care Services A medical school provides its medical students with timely access to needed diagnostic, preventive, and therapeutic health services at sites in reasonable proximity to the locations of their required educational experiences and has policies and procedures in place that permit students to be excused from these experiences to seek needed care.
12.5 Non-involvement of Providers of Student Health Services in Student Assessment/Location of Student Health Records The health professionals who provide health services, including psychiatric/psychological counseling, to a medical student have no involvement in the academic assessment or promotion of the medical student receiving those services. A medical school ensures that medical student health records are maintained in accordance with legal requirements for security, privacy, confidentiality, and accessibility.

Key Stressors in Medical School that Can Impact Students' Well-Being

Lack of Sleep

Medical students are often surprised to find that work, clinical duties, and studying take up a substantial part of their day. In a time-limited 24-hour day, when precious hours are needed to study for an exam or to pre-round on patients for the following day, students tend to sacrifice sleep to make up some of the needed time. Soon, the 7 hours of recommended sleep [3] is no longer the norm, with students resorting to 4 and 5 hours per evening in an effort to accomplish all of their other work.

Research suggests, however, that 4–5 hours of sleep and consistent sleep deprivation have significant consequences for medical students including "nodding off" while driving, feeling more overwhelmed and "down," and expressing greater dissatisfaction with their quality of life [16]. Poor sleep has consequences for the public at large, including weight gain and obesity, diabetes, hypertension, heart disease and stroke, depression, impaired immune function, increased pain, impaired performance, increased errors, and greater risk of accidents [3].

Poor sleep (defined as less than 6 hours) is associated with elevated risk of depression in the first months of internship and medical errors in residents [17], and concern has been expressed by the psychiatric community that the continued sleep deficits and poor sleep habits that begin in medical school may continue into training and practice, with compelling negative consequences for the physician workforce and the health of the public [14].

Tip
Students should aim for 7 hours of sleep per night or "restful" sleep that ensures optimal performance and concentration and should practice good sleep hygiene and remove electronic devices from their sleeping space.

Tip
Students who try to learn when exhausted don't perform well. Sleeping for even a few hours and then returning to studying can be far more effective than studying while exhausted.

Lack of Connection

Socialization and connectedness are critical to ongoing well-being. Medical school can be a time when students, taxed with multiple competing demands, draw inward and devote a disproportionate amount of time to studying at the expense of socializing with family and friends. However, a significantly greater risk of depression has been associated with inadequate support from family, friends, and other medical students [35]. It is therefore important for medical students to connect to their peer group and to stay in touch with family and friends. To facilitate this sense of connectedness, medical schools should foster both small and large group activities that go beyond simple learning and offer an opportunity to investigate shared interests, hobbies, and future goals.

Medical schools can also provide space for sharing and support. When medical students are given the opportunity to share struggles and approaches to maintaining wellness with their peers in a supportive and safe space, they discover that they are not alone. The realization that others have similar challenges, feel overwhelmed, or struggle with depression or anxiety can normalize these feelings. Cohorts often have a positive impact on peers' help-seeking behaviors. When one student seeks mental health services and has a positive outcome, it may influence others' decisions about seeking help.

Tip
Provide students with the opportunity to share their experiences. Often, a second- or third-year student discussing the benefits of mental health services can be a great motivator for first-year students, still navigating the medical school environment, to seek help.

Lack of Exercise

The same demands on students' time often lead to a decrease in exercise. In a recent single-site study, decreased exercise frequency was significantly correlated with lower professional efficacy [36]. While the benefits of exercise are fully covered in Chap. 5 of this book, it is understandable how the cascade of events (increased need to study leading to deficits in sleep, exercise, and social connectedness) can quickly contribute to a decrease in overall wellness leading to negative psychological and physical effects.

Relentless Pace

The curriculum of medical school can feel all-consuming and unforgiving. Students compare medical school to trying to drink water from a firehose. The pace of the first year or two of medical school is often based in lecture halls and small group rooms. It tends to be fast; the breaks are few; knowledge builds upon prior knowledge: it might feel like one can never catch a break. Students with mental health issues who are struggling and who might need to take time off frequently avoid doing so, because missing even a short period of time can put one behind. Medical schools can help students put their mental health first by developing a few alternative paths to completing coursework in the first 2 years. Allowing students to step out and re-enter the following year at the same time in the curriculum, having planned remediation periods for the didactic years (e.g., over Thanksgiving and Christmas break, summer), allows students to "catch up" and catch their breath when a mental health challenges place them off track.

Students who require time off in the clerkship year can often step out of a clerkship, allowing them a 2–8-week break depending on the rotation. Allowing the students to resume or retake the clerkship at a later date allows them to seek the mental health help they need in a timely manner. While stepping out might lessen some of the student's elective time, it may enable the student to stay on track toward graduation.

> **Tip**
> The first-year curriculum, while challenging, often includes a more predictable and flexible schedule. It is the *perfect time* for a consultation and possible treatment if a student has any mental health concerns or finds themselves developing psychological symptoms.

> **Tip**
> Students who require hospitalization in the clinical year may be able to step out of rotation and re-enter without causing major disruption to their plan of study or graduation. Students should be aware of this option to encourage help-seeking behavior for students in acute distress.

High-Stakes Environment

The high-stakes environment of medicine is well-documented. Within medical education there are specific times of higher stress, for example, the time period leading up to the US Medical Licensing Examination (USMLE) Step 1, the transition from the preclinical curriculum to the clerkship year, and the time devoted to the National Resident Matching Program, commonly known as "the match." In a recent commentary, the authors lament about the impact of the Step 1 examination saying, "it is disconcerting that the test preoccupies so much of students' attention with attendant substantial costs (in time and money) and mental and emotional anguish" (Ref. [29], pg. 12). Scores from the Step 1 are often used in screening applicants for residency. In some cases, they are used to determine, or limit, a student's future prospects for specialization and matching. Many of the more competitive residencies (e.g., orthopedic surgery, dermatology, ophthalmology, otolaryngology, etc.) maintain high threshold scores for consideration despite the lack of predictive value for future success [22]. Prober and colleagues also discuss the unintended consequences in the use of such high stakes on mental health and wellness. They cite the high incidence of burnout, depression, and suicidal ideation and note that "an undue emphasis on USMLE Step 1, driven by its common role in screening for residency selection, contributes unnecessarily to this stress."

These very real consequences are recounted in commentaries like "Murky Water" by Catherine Lapedis [18], where the author discusses her emotional exhaustion as a result of taking the USMLE Step 1, and how her school described the exam as deciding, "who would succeed ….who would choose their specialty….who would live in the same location as their loved ones and who would be separated."

This commentary, while sadly recounting the stressors that unnecessarily added to the Step 1 experience for the author, also conveys the most extreme impacts of the Step 1 on mental health. One of the authors' peers who also received her score that fateful day took her life, as recounted by the author, "Minutes later, Sarah called 911; reported, "I'm going to kill myself"; and hung up. She was gone before the ambulance arrived. Next to her body lay her laptop displaying the results of her examination. She had failed by one point."

> **Tip**
> Medical schools should espouse a balanced approach to the Step 1 exam. There are students who fail, retake the exam and pass, and go on to be happy, productive physicians.

> **Tip**
> Remediation and support teams should be more robust immediately preceding and following the Step 1 administration. Schools should be aware of students who fail in advance and reach out to offer support and future-oriented plans for remediation that focus on positive outcomes. As noted above, students should have information on hand for the suicide prevention hotline.

Distinguishing Between Adjustment and Anxiety/Depression

For many students, differentiating between adjustment to medical education and the beginnings of episodic or chronic anxiety and depression can be difficult. It is important to be aware of the signs and symptoms associated with the onset of anxiety and depression and distinguish these from the anticipated adjustments to medical school (see Table 2.2). At the first sign of clinical anxiety or depression, students should seek counsel from a medical professional. Addressing these issues early in medical education and early in presentation of symptoms not only lessens the duration of the student's stress but also reduces the overall impact on one's education. Students who engage in cognitive-behavioral therapy (as noted above) can begin learning skills and tools to improve mental health in the first few sessions.

> **Tip**
> When students find themselves more anxious and tense, they should ask for objective feedback and review the table on adjustment vs. symptoms of anxiety/depression.

TABLE 2.2 Comparison of adjustment and anxiety/depression

Anticipated adjustments	Symptoms of anxiety/depression
Slight decrease or increase in sleep	Significant increase or decrease in sleep
Feelings of being overwhelmed that fade quickly (within the hour)	Feelings of being overwhelmed or impending doom that do not subside quickly or impair your ability to focus or study
Tearful and temporary responses to negative clinical events (death of a patient, severe trauma in clinic)	Emotional lability, panic attacks, crying that does not subside within a brief period of time
Reduction in social time with friends, but still maintaining contact (in person, by phone, facetime, text) with family and friends	Continuous decline in time with friends and lack of contact with family and friends (no communication for many weeks)

Tip

Schools should offer students objective feedback when they notice a change in behavior or mood. Schools can review Table 2.2 with students, helping them identify whether their symptoms are due to adjustment or if there are reasonable concerns about anxiety/depression.

Ideally, medical students should aim to care for their overall well-being as they navigate medical education. As noted above, this includes getting plenty of sleep, maintaining an exercise routine, and tending to their mental health. For students with a history of mental health challenges, it is important to connect with a provider and establish care proactively.

Disability and Medical Education: Navigating the Landscape

There are times when a mental health issue rises to the level of disability. When this occurs, students may be eligible for protections under the Americans with Disabilities Act [2] and may be eligible for reasonable accommodations under Section 504 of the Rehabilitation Act [32]. Most post-secondary institutions—including medical schools—are required to provide students with appropriate academic adjustments and auxiliary aids and services. Medical schools, however, are not required to make adjustments or provide aids or services that would result in a fundamental alteration of the program or impose an undue financial or administrative burden on the institution.

One might ask how a well-qualified student in medical school could simultaneously be considered a person with a disability. A qualified student with a disability is a student with a disability who meets the academic and technical standards for admission or participation in the institution's educational program or activity.

> **Example**
> A medical student with bipolar disorder was recently started on a new medication for depressive symptoms and is doing well psychologically. However, the student has been noticing side effects that include drowsiness and slowed processing. This student finds that the side effects of the medication are now causing significant barriers in medical school regarding finishing exams in the allotted time. The student remains a qualified medical student meeting the technical standards, but due to the disabling impact of medication, he/she requires an accommodation, in this case, 25% additional time to complete his/her exams.

Importantly, students with psychological disabilities often remain highly qualified for medical school and a career in medicine. These students have the abilities outlined in the technical standards of medical schools and are capable of learning and applying clinical knowledge and providing excellent care to their patients. The disability-related barriers that exist are often a result of the medical school environment. By removing or attenuating the barriers, students are able to display their knowledge and abilities. In our example case, a student, as a result of medication, may find that it takes longer to read questions on an exam or that the questions need to be read multiple times before they can fully process the information. In a time-limited scenario, this student may face a distinct barrier to the exam: time. The student has the clinical knowledge to answer the questions correctly but might run out of time due to the functional limitations (slowed processing or interrupted concentration) that result from the side effects of their medication. In this instance, the student could be both a qualified medical student and a person with a disability who is eligible for reasonable accommodations (extra time) under the ADA and Section 504 of the Rehabilitation Act.

Psychological disabilities are only one of the categories of disability. Others include learning, chronic health, physical, and sensory disability. Many students may find themselves at the intersection multiple categories.

Example
A student who is diagnosed with a chronic health condition—for example, an autoimmune disease—may find that because of his/her primary diagnosis, he/she experiences a co-occurring psychological disability, like depression or anxiety. In this case, the student may already be receiving accommodations for the autoimmune disease (e.g., ability to take breaks on the wards, intentional breaks between clinical rotations) but may also require a release from clinic to attend appointments with their therapist due to the secondary disability of anxiety.

TABLE 2.3 Common accommodations for psychological disabilities in clinical settings

Functional limitation	Accommodation
Slowed processing	1. Dragon dictate: speech-to-text technology to assist with charting 2. Assigned patients for presenting
Difficulty with concentration	1. Smart pens for recording patient intake 2. Reminders set on watch to direct use of time 3. Noise-cancelling headphones for charting
Panic attacks	1. Laminated list of how to present patient worn on badge (to facilitate ease of reference) 2. Pre-assigned patients for presenting 3. Ability to take 10-minute breaks throughout the day to meditate and practice calming techniques 4. Release from clinic for weekly therapy appointments
Anxiety	1. Release from clinic to go to weekly mental health appointments 2. Request clinical rotations in geographical areas that allow continued therapy

Below are some of the most commonly recommended accommodations for students with psychological disabilities in clinical settings (see Table 2.3) and in clerkship placements (see Table 2.4) [23, 26]. This list is not meant to be exhaustive and may vary between Undergraduate Medical Education (UME) and Graduate Medical Education (GME) programs.

Tip
Students with psychological disabilities that impact functioning should seek accommodations in medical school and on high-stakes exams.

TABLE 2.4 Common accommodations for psychological disabilities for clerkship placements

Need	Potential accommodation
Weekly appointments	1. Release from clinical duties to attend appointments. Time missed to be made up on alternative day
Continuous sleep	1. Weekend day call in lieu of overnight call 2. Hard stop on wards by 10 pm
Getting to the clinical site: parking/driving	1. Designated parking or access to parking space to allow student to leave and return quickly from appointments 2. Placement at clinical sites within a specified radius of a student's primary provider's location to facilitate weekly appointments
Clerkship order scheduling	1. Ordering of clerkship to allow for break time between physically taxing rotations (surgery/medicine/ob-gyn) 2. Scheduling of clerkships to provide equal distribution of physically taxing rotations (e.g., avoiding medicine and surgery back to back)
Prior treatment at the site	1. Thoughtful placement into clerkship sites to avoid having student rotate at locations where they were admitted or evaluated (e.g., through ED, in-patient psychiatry, ICU)

Institutions can take several steps to mitigate the impact of a mental health-related disability. In keeping with LCME guidance [19], medical schools should release medical students for mental health-related appointments. Many schools formalize this release through the dean of students, the disability support office, or the counseling services offices as a disability-related accommodation. Some schools choose to embed protected time into the curriculum for all students to attend to their various needs. Others maintain blanket policies that all students are allowed to miss a set number of hours weekly to engage in mental health or wellness activities.

> **Tip**
> Medical schools should consider embedding protected time into the curriculum for all students to attend to medical or mental health needs.

LCME guidance also requires that schools have medical care available in close proximity to the clinical site. Medical schools can accommodate a student by ensuring that the student's clinical rotations are relatively close to their mental health provider. Medical students benefit from continuity of care with their provider and by ensuring they make their weekly or biweekly appointments. For schools that are unable to place students nearby, they may consider providing a private and protected (reserved, quiet, no traffic) space for students to meet with their provider by phone or video conference. Indeed, schools might consider having all mental health providers become capable of providing telepsychiatry or teletherapy sessions during all years, but especially in the clinical years as an extension of the traditional services offered during the didactic portion of medical school. This allows for continuity of care in a less logistically challenging format.

> **Tip**
> Medical schools should explore ways of utilizing telepsychiatry/teletherapy, when clinically appropriate, to enable this generation of tech-savvy students, often pressed for time or at faraway locations, the chance to get the mental health care they need.

In 2018, the University of California, San Francisco, and the Association of American Medical Colleges released a special report titled *Accessibility, Inclusion, and Action in Medical Education: Lived Experiences of Learners and Physicians with Disabilities* [24]. The report chronicles the lived experience of students, resident, and physicians with disabilities. Throughout the report, and in particular in the report's appendix, the authors offer recommendations for programs and students. Medical schools and residency programs should review this report to ensure that their practices align with the considerations offered in the report appendices.

Programs should also ensure that a qualified individual with experience in the ADA leads a robust and legally mandated interactive process for determining eligibility for services and reasonable accommodations. The 2018 report from The University of California, San Francisco (UCSF) and the The Association of American Medical Colleges (AAMC) outlines the interactive process in detail and provides thoughtful considerations for medical schools and residency programs engaging with the disability process. As well, the AAMC offers a webinar about supporting students with psychological disabilities in medical school and provides detailed recommendations about leaves of absence, release from overnight call, reasonable accommodations, and decision-making [26].

Sharing Experiences

When medical students are given the opportunity to share struggles and approaches to maintaining wellness with their peers in a supportive and safe space, they discover that they are not alone. The realization that others have similar struggles, feel overwhelmed, or struggle with depression or anxiety can normalize these feelings for other medical students who may incorrectly feel that they are alone in these feelings. Cohorts often have a positive impact on peers' help-seeking behaviors. When one student seeks mental health or disability services and has a positive outcome, it may influence others' decisions about seeking help.

Leaves of Absence

In some instances, students experiencing a mental health crisis may need to take a leave of absence (LOA). Taking a leave of absence should be an easy process, requiring only a physician signature stating that the leave is medically necessary. No information about the diagnosis, planned treatment, medication, or therapy should be requested. Medical schools should ensure that their LOA process does not serve as a deterrent by requesting detailed information about a student's mental health or requiring students to gain multiple signatures from faculty or administrators as part of the process. Students who see the LOA as an additional barrier or who have to disclose personal sensitive information about their mental health may "push through" rather than disclose a mental health issue if they are concerned about having to inform a medical school official who might be involved in evaluation, grading, recommendations, or promotion.

Confidentiality

Maintaining confidentiality of student mental health records and status as a person with a disability is paramount. If students do not trust the program, they will not disclose mental health challenges and are less likely to engage in help-seeking behavior. Medical schools should ensure that policies for registering with disability services, seeking mental health services, or taking a leave of absence address confidentiality or privacy of information.

Disability Insurance

While students are not required to take out disability insurance, medical schools are required by the LCME to offer the option to all students (see Table 2.5). Disability insurance can be used in multiple ways but is most often put into effect

TABLE 2.5 LCME element 12.6

12.6 Student Health and Disability Insurance
A medical school ensures that health insurance and disability insurance are available to each medical student and that health insurance is also available to each medical student's dependents.

when a student needs to take an extended leave of absence (6 or more months). In the event of a disability-related need to suspend or discontinue medical education, insurance provides a low-cost protection and can serve as a source of income to pay living expenses and help with loan repayment in the event of disability. Costs are low for enrolling in disability insurance, and the average insurance coverage offers generous support to students who are out of school for any period of time due to disability. The authors recommend that all schools provide disability insurance coverage for all medical students, regardless of medical history.

> **Tip**
> Medical schools should provide disability insurance for all students. The very small investment provides excellent coverage, which may be the catalyst to ensuring students take a LOA and seek help when needed.

Concluding Thoughts

Medical school is hard. One in four medical students will experience a mental health issue. Depression rates for medical students are higher than age-matched peers. Over 10% of medical students think about suicide, the rate of burnout is 50%, and leaders in the medical community believe we have hit a crisis level.

Something about medical school correlates with worsening mental health and well-being. What is it? We should look at the culture of medicine. Students hear stories about physicians who place their needs behind those of their patients, and they strive to become them. The selfless and noble physician is heralded as the ideal. How many of us have been regaled by tales of our physician forbearers who have worked longer, harder, and with barely a day off?

If students are struggling in any way, they can feel alienated when they sense that they might not be living up to that mythic ideal. Medical students are perceptive, and they pick up on stigmas. They worry that having mental health issues could affect their chances of residency and future success. They do not want to be perceived as weak. Thus, it is important that students be taught, mentored, and supported by faculty, staff, and educational leadership who understand this current environment, are mindful of the mental health issues of medical students, and are aware that these conditions can benefit from treatment, mitigating measures, reasonable accommodations, and guidance from medical education organizations.

We hope that this chapter serves as a valuable overview of the state of mental health of medical students today. We hope that medical schools use this as a guide to improve the medical education experience for all students. We must not only help the medical student in front of us, but we must also reach those students who may be suffering in silence.

Appendix A: Top 20 Tips for Medical Students and Administrators

Tip
Students should seek treatment during the first year of medical school for specific phobias. These phobias can limit their opportunities and they are treatable.

Tip
Students who experience anxiety around presenting students or clinical encounters with patients may find relief using the basic principles of systematic desensitization, whereby schools expose the student to incremental patient encounters or patient presentations using a simulation lab and standardized patients.

Tip
Students who experience anxiety while engaging in small group discussions or presentations should reach out to counseling for assistance. Performance can improve, and students will enjoy the experience.

Tip
Students who experience panic attacks while on the wards can use bathroom stalls as safe space to regroup and meditate or medicate. Bathrooms are usually close by when students feel an impending attack, and social graces dictate that others do not place critical inquiry on time spent in a restroom, giving the student a short, but much needed and socially accepted reprieve.

Tip
Students who lose the ability to enjoy things that usually bring them pleasure may be experiencing anhedonia, one of the key symptoms of major depression.

Tip
Medical students with a history of mental health concerns or treatment should get connected to a mental health provider as soon as they arrive at school. Establishing care and a relationship with a provider is imperative, even when things are going well.

Tip
Students having thoughts of suicide should have access to an emergency contact person at the school, and the National Suicide Prevention Hotline should be posted in multiple, easy-to-access locations (online, student handbook, badge stickers). The NSPH number is 1–800–273-8255 and is staffed 24/7.

Tip
Students should aim for 7 hours of sleep per night or "restful" sleep that ensures optimal performance and concentration and should practice good sleep hygiene and remove electronic devices from their sleeping space.

Tip
Students who try to learn when exhausted don't perform well. Sleeping for even a few hours and then returning to studying can be far more effective than studying while exhausted.

Tip
Provide students with the opportunity to share their experiences. Often, a second- or third-year student discussing the benefits of mental health services can be a great motivator for first-year students, still navigating the medical school environment, to seek help.

Tip
The first-year curriculum, while challenging, often includes a more predictable and flexible schedule. It is the *perfect time* for a consultation and possible treatment if a student has any mental health concerns or finds themselves developing psychological symptoms.

Tip
Students who require hospitalization in the clinical year may be able to step out of rotation and re-enter without causing major disruption to their plan of study or graduation. Students should be aware of this option to encourage help-seeking behavior for students in acute distress.

Tip
Medical schools should espouse a balanced approach to the Step 1 exam. There are students who fail, retake the exam and pass, and go on to be happy, productive physicians.

Tip
Remediation and support teams should be more robust immediately preceding and following the Step 1 administration. Schools should be aware of students who fail in advance and reach out to offer support and future-oriented plans for remediation that focus on positive outcomes. As noted above, students should have information on hand for the suicide prevention hotline.

Tip
When students find themselves more anxious and tense, they should ask for objective feedback and review the table on adjustment vs. symptoms of anxiety/depression.

Tip
Schools should offer students objective feedback when they notice a change in behavior or mood. Schools can review Table 2.2 with students, helping them identify whether their symptoms are due to adjustment or if there are reasonable concerns about anxiety/depression.

Tip
Students with psychological disabilities that impact functioning should seek accommodations in medical school and on high-stakes exams.

> **Tip**
> Medical schools should consider embedding protected time into the curriculum for all students to attend to medical or mental health needs.

> **Tip**
> Medical schools should explore ways of utilizing tele-psychiatry/teletherapy, when clinically appropriate, to enable this generation of tech-savvy students, often pressed for time or at faraway locations, the chance to get the mental health care they need.

> **Tip**
> Medical schools should consider maintaining disability insurance for all students. The very small investment provides excellent coverage, which may be the catalyst to ensuring students take a LOA and seek help when needed.

References

1. American Foundation for Suicide Prevention. Ten facts about physician suicide and mental health. http://afsp.org/wp-content/uploads/2016/11/ten-facts-about-physician-suicide.pdf (2016). Accessed 31 Dec 2017.
2. Americans with Disabilities Act of 1990, Pub. L. No. 101-336, § 2, 104 Stat. 328 (1991).
3. Badr MS, Belenky G, Bliwise DL, Buxton OM, Buysse D, Dinges DF, et al. Recommended amount of sleep for a healthy adult: a joint consensus statement of the American Academy of

Sleep Medicine and Sleep Research Society. J Clin Sleep Med. 2015;11(06):591–2.

4. Blacker J, Lewis P, Swintak C, Bostwick M, Rackley J. Medical student suicide rates: a systematic review of the historical and international literature. Acad Med. 2018; https://doi.org/10.1097/ACM.0000000000002430.

5. Center C, Davis M, Detre T, Ford DE, Hansbrough W, Hendin H, Laszlo J, Litts DA, Mann J, Mansky PA, Michels R, Miles SH, Proujansky R, Reynolds CF 3rd, Silverman MM. Confronting depression and suicide in physicians. JAMA. 2003;289(23):3161–6. https://doi.org/10.1001/jama.289.23.3161.

6. Dyrbye N, Thomas R, Shanafelt D. Systematic review of depression, anxiety, and other indicators of psychological distress among U.S. and Canadian medical students. Acad Med. 2006;81(4):354–73. https://doi.org/10.1097/00001888-200604000-00009.

7. Dyrbye L, Thomas M, Massie F, Power D, Eacker A, Harper W, et al. Burnout and suicidal ideation among U.S. medical students. Ann Intern Med. 2008;149(5):334–33441. https://doi.org/10.7326/0003-4819-149-5-200809020-01003.

8. Dyrbye L, Massie F, Eacker A, Harper W, Power D, Durning S, et al. Relationship between burnout and professional conduct and attitudes among medical students. JAMA. 2010;304(11):1173–80. https://doi.org/10.1001/jama.2010.1318.

9. Dyrbye N, Thomas R, Power V, Durning S, Moutier W, Massie A, et al. Burnout and serious thoughts of dropping out of medical school: a multi-institutional study. Acad Med. 2010;85(1):94–102. https://doi.org/10.1097/ACM.0b013e3181c46aad.

10. Dyrbye N, West P, Satele D, Boone D, Tan D, Sloan D, Shanafelt D. Burnout among U.S. medical students, residents, and early career physicians relative to the general U.S. population. Acad Med. 2014;89(3):443–51. https://doi.org/10.1097/ACM.0000000000000134.

11. Dzau V, Kirch D, Nasca T. To care is human – collectively confronting the clinician-burnout crisis. N Engl J Med. 2018;378(4):312–4. https://doi.org/10.1056/NEJMp1715127.

12. Givens JL, Tjia J. Depressed medical students' use of mental health services and barriers to use. Acad Med. 2002;77(9):918–21.

13. Gold K, Sen A, Schwenk T. Details on suicide among US physicians: data from the National Violent Death Reporting System. Gen Hosp Psychiatry. 2013;35(1):45–9. https://doi.org/10.1016/j.genhosppsych.2012.08.005.

14. Grady F, Roberts LW. Sleep deprived and overwhelmed: sleep behaviors of medical students in the USA. Acad Psychiatry. 2017;41:661. https://doi.org/10.1007/s40596-017-0804-3.

15. Jackson R, Shanafelt D, Hasan V, Satele N, Dyrbye N. Burnout and alcohol abuse/dependence among U.S. medical students. Acad Med. 2016;91(9):1251–6. https://doi.org/10.1097/ACM.0000000000001138.

16. Johnson KM, Simon N, Wicks M, Barr K, O'Connor K, Schaad D. Amount of sleep, daytime sleepiness, hazardous driving, and quality of life of second year medical students. Acad Psychiatry. 2017;41(5):669–73.

17. Kalmbach DA, Arnedt JT, Song PX, Guille C, Sen S. Sleep disturbance and short sleep as risk factors for depression and perceived medical errors in first-year residents. Sleep. 2017;40(3)

18. Lapedis CJ. Murky water. Ann Intern Med. 2018;169:415–6. https://doi.org/10.7326/M18-1398.

19. Liaison Committee on Medical Education (LCME). Functions and structure of a medical school: standards for accreditation of medical education programs leading to the MD degree. Washington, DC/Chicago: LCME; 2016. Effective 1 July 2017. http://lcme.org/publications. Accessed 25 Dec 2018

20. Linzer M, Manwell L, Williams E, Bobula J, Brown R, Varkey A, et al. Working conditions in primary care: physician reactions and care quality. Ann Intern Med. 2009;151(1):28–36., W6–9. https://doi.org/10.7326/0003-4819-151-1-200907070-00006.

21. Ludwig A, Burton W, Weingarten J, Milan F, Myers D, Kligler B. Depression and stress amongst undergraduate medical students. BMC Med Educ. 2015;15(1):141. https://doi.org/10.1186/s12909-015-0425-z.

22. McGaghie WC, Cohen ER, Wayne DB. Are United States medical licensing exam step 1 and 2 scores valid measures for postgraduate medical residency selection decisions? Acad Med. 2011;86(1):48–52. https://doi.org/10.1097/ACM.0b013e3181ffacdb.

23. Meeks L, Jain N. The guide to assisting students with disabilities: equal access in health science and professional education. New York: Springer Publishing Company; 2016.

24. Meeks LM, Jain NR. Accessibility, inclusion, and action in medical education: lived experiences of learners and physicians with disabilities. Washington, DC: Association of American Medical Colleges; 2018.

25. Monroe S, Simons A. Diathesis-stress theories in the context of life stress research: implications for the depressive disorders. Psychol Bull. 1991;110(3):406–25.
26. Murray J, Papdakis M, Meeks L. Supporting students with psychological disabilities in medical school. [Webinar]. Association of American Medical Colleges Webinar Series on working with students with disabilities (2016, March 10th). Retrieved from https://www.aamc.org/members/gsa/pdopportunities/454436/studentswithpsychologicaldisabilities.html. 4 Jan 2019.
27. National Academy of Medicine. (2018). Clinician resilience and well-being – National Academy of Medicine. [online] Available at: https://nam.edu/clinicianwellbeing/. Accessed 1 Jan 2018.
28. National Institute of Mental Health. Mental health information: statistics. (2017). https://www.nimh.nih.gov/health/statistics/mental-illness.shtml. Accessed 1 Dec 2018.
29. Prober G, Kolars C, First R, Melnick E. A plea to reassess the role of United States medical licensing examination step 1 scores in residency selection. Acad Med. 2016;91(1):12–5. https://doi.org/10.1097/ACM.0000000000000855.
30. Rotenstein L, Ramos M, Torre M, Segal J, Peluso M, Guille C, et al. Prevalence of depression, depressive symptoms, and suicidal ideation among medical students: a systematic review and meta-analysis. JAMA. 2016;316(21):2214–36. https://doi.org/10.1001/jama.2016.17324.
31. Schernhammer ES, Colditz GA. Suicide rates among physicians: a quantitative and gender assessment (meta-analysis). Am J Psychiatry. 2004;161(12):2295–302. https://doi.org/10.1176/appi.ajp.161.12.2295.
32. Section 504 of the Rehabilitation Act of 1973, Pub. L. No. 93-112, §701 (1973).
33. Shanafelt T, Oreskovich M, Sloan J, West C, Satele D, Sotile A, et al. Burnout and satisfaction with work-life balance among US physicians relative to the general US population. Arch Intern Med. 2012;172(18):1377–85. https://doi.org/10.1001/archinternmed.2012.3199.
34. Shanafelt T, Hasan O, Dyrbye L, Sinsky C, Satele D, Sloan J, West C. Changes in burnout and satisfaction with work-life balance in physicians and the general US working population between 2011 and 2014. Mayo Clin Proc. 2015;90(12):1600–13. https://doi.org/10.1016/j.mayocp.2015.08.023.

35. Thompson G, Mcbride R, Hosford C, Halaas G. Resilience among medical students: the role of coping style and social support. Teach Learn Med. 2016;28(2):174–82. https://doi.org/10.108 0/10401334.2016.1146611.
36. Wolf M, Rosenstock J. Inadequate sleep and exercise associated with burnout and depression among medical students. Acad Psychiatry. 2017;41(2):174–9. https://doi.org/10.1007/ s40596-016-0526-y.
37. Yaghmour A, Brigham P, Richter S, Miller C, Philibert J, Baldwin J, Nasca J. Causes of death of residents in ACGME-accredited programs 2000 through 2014: implications for the learning environment. Acad Med. 2017;92(7):976–83. https://doi.org/10.1097/ ACM.0000000000001736.

Chapter 3
Medical Students and Substance Use Disorders

Kristopher A. Kast and Jonathan D. Avery

Medical students—and the medical community as a whole—are often thought to be relatively protected from substance use disorders (SUDs) due to increased knowledge about the harm of addictive behaviors. Medical students, however, have been shown to use more alcohol and other substances than similar, age-matched peers in several studies [5, 6, 14, 18, 22, 32, 40]. Addiction is a complex neuropsychiatric disorder with heritable risk, conserved neuropathology, chronic relapsing course, and multiple effective treatment modalities [27]. As with many psychiatric diagnoses, addiction spares no group of individuals. Substance use disorders (SUDs) in medical students and physicians were historically viewed as unethical behavior subject to severe disciplinary action, until the American Medical Association advocated a medical model for assessment and treatment of impaired physicians in a landmark publication [41].

———

K. A. Kast (✉)
New York Presbyterian Hospital/Weill Cornell Medical College,
New York, NY, USA
e-mail: Kak9100@nyp.org

J. D. Avery
Cornell University Weill Cornell Medical College,
New York, NY, USA
e-mail: Joa9070@med.cornell.edu

© Springer Nature Switzerland AG 2019
D. Zappetti, J. D. Avery (eds.), *Medical Student Well-Being*,
https://doi.org/10.1007/978-3-030-16558-1_3

TABLE 3.1 Tips for medical students and faculty

Medical students	Faculty
Learn to identify problematic substance use early (for yourself and your peers)	Learn to recognize the signs of substance use in students
Seek treatment immediately or intervene for peers using available resources	Intervene for students immediately so that they can take advantage of early treatment
Be mindful of the stigma of substance use disorders as a barrier to care	Be mindful of the stigma of substance use disorders as a barrier to care
Familiarize yourself with resources for impaired students at your medical school	Familiarize yourself with resources for impaired students at your medical school and with your state-specific legal requirements around reporting and referral to care

This paradigm shift conceptualized SUD as an illness and increased access to SUD treatment for impaired medical students and physicians. Here, we discuss the complex relationship between medical student populations, substances, stigma-based barriers to care, effective treatment options, and important concurrent safeguards to public safety. Table 3.1 provides some simple tips for students and faculty.

Substance Use Patterns

The lifetime prevalence of any substance use disorder (SUD) among physicians is 8–15%, with a point prevalence of 2–3.8% [10, 16, 26, 33]. A similar point prevalence of 0.6–3.3% for self-perceived problematic substance use was reported in a large medical student population, with 2.3–6.3% of medical students reporting attempts to reduce their substance use [32].

Alcohol use disorder is the most prevalent SUD among physicians and medical students [16, 22, 32]. There is also a more recent rise in cannabis use disorder [10]. Among medical students, 91–96% report using any alcohol, and 22.7–26% report using cannabis in medical school [5, 32]. A large subgroup, from 30% to 70%, report binge alcohol use, consuming five or more drinks in one sitting [5, 32]. Prescription and non-prescription stimulant, opioid, sedative/hypnotic, hallucinogen, and tobacco use disorders also occur [20, 22, 32]. While most medical students report reducing substance use during medical school, a significant minority report increasing use [32].

Genetic loading for SUD is the greatest risk factor for development of SUD in medical students and physicians [17]. Risk of problematic alcohol use among medical students is increased with comorbid burnout, depression, single marital status, younger age, and high educational debt [25]. Use of opioids and sedative/hypnotics also occurs in medical school, both from prescription and non-prescription sources, but the risk appears to increase during residency training with the onset of prescribing privileges; these physicians report initiating self-prescribing for "self-treatment" rather than recreation—highlighting a unique iatrogenic risk among trainees [24].

Higher academic performance and narcissistic or obsessive-compulsive personality traits are also associated with some degree of risk for SUD among medical students [15–17]. Further, excessive alcohol use among medical students was reported to have no impact on clinical rotation performance [16]. This is consistent with the hypothesis that deterioration in the workplace is a late finding among physicians and medical students with SUD, contributing to a troubling delay in SUD treatment [9, 10, 12].

Reported mortality rates for physicians with SUD range from 3.7% to 18% in different samples, with deaths due to overdose, medical complications of SUD, and suicide [19, 29, 44]. Alcohol intoxication, SUD diagnosis, and self-prescription of medication are all associated with documented physician suicides [16]. Additional risks include legal repercussions (e.g., driving while intoxicated) and increased interpersonal conflict at home and in the work-place [30]. These risks have been less clearly defined in the medical student population, with notably fewer suicides among medical students (compared to age-matched controls) and none associated with reported SUD [45] however, this may only reflect a relative delay in the risk until the medical student with SUD has graduated.

Addiction, Impairment, and Access to Care

Functional impairment and an SUD diagnosis are distinct but overlapping categories [36, 37]. The window of opportunity between illness onset and impairment may be more than 6 years in the physician population [9, 10, 12]. Untreated SUD typically progresses to impairment, but early identification and intervention may prevent impairment and lead to recovery. However, potent barriers limit early referral of affected medical students.

Barriers to care-seeking in medical students with early SUD include prevalent denial-based unconscious defenses (i.e., unconsciously motivated repression of conscious awareness of the problem behavior), stigma-motivated conscious concealment (i.e., knowingly hiding problem behavior due to feared social or professional consequences), aversion to assuming the patient role, difficulty obtaining leave from medical school during treatment (or reluctance to remove oneself from a peer cohort), and fear of disciplinary action from medical schools or licensing boards [37].

The unintended consequence of a punitive approach to medical student (and physician) impairment — once common among medical schools and state licensing boards — is delayed treatment. Ill medical students and physicians are unwilling to risk the far-reaching consequences of removal from medical school or permanently suspended medical licensure, and concerned peers and faculty may similarly balk at these high stakes when considering intervention. Among a large sample of medical students, 49–53% indicated unwillingness to report an impaired peer, preferring to maintain confidentiality and encourage the peer to seek help [42]. This culture of secrecy and shame promotes treatment avoidance and progression to functional impairment, with resulting exposure of the public to unidentified and untreated impaired physicians or physicians-in-training [37].

To address this issue, the American Medical Association and the Federation of State Medical Boards advocate for access to voluntary tracks for medical students and physicians with SUD to receive confidential treatment while maintaining adequate safeguards protecting public safety. Medical school mental health programs and physician health programs (PHPs) are the mechanism by which evaluation, referral to treatment, and subsequent monitoring for stability of recovery typically occur in the United States.

PHPs may be underutilized by medical students and medical schools. Rates of medical student enrollment in PHPs are infrequently reported and range from 2% to 7% of total medical professional enrollment [8, 43]. PHPs manage the evaluation, treatment, and post-treatment monitoring of medical students (and other healthcare professionals) who have signed voluntary contracts to participate in the program. Medical students are either self-referred or referred by colleagues or medical school administrators to PHPs, which are organized by the state medical board or medical societies. PHPs do not provide medical services; they are an independent third party that enrolls and refers patients to specialist treatment and provides post-treatment relapse monitoring for up to 5 years to ensure stability of recovery [11, 35]. PHPs allow competing ethical obligations—preservation of public safety and protection of patients' right to treatment and recovery—to be simultaneously safeguarded through a system largely separate from the legal-professional governing bodies. Self-referred medical students are usually able to participate confidentially.

Identifying the Medical Student
with a Substance Use Disorder

Medical students' initial presentations with SUD vary widely in severity. The most common presentations include self-identification of risky use or early use disorder, non-specific abnormal workplace or academic behavior, poor or incomplete documentation or assignment completion, absenteeism, witnessed substance use or intoxication in the hospital or medical school campus (varying in severity from odor of alcohol on the breath to observed intravenous injection of hospital opioids), and death by accidental or intentional overdose [14, 19, 22]. Notably, some medical students with SUD may be more impaired when the substance is absent (i.e., in a state of withdrawal or craving and preoccupation) than when it is present [26].

It is an ethical obligation to report impaired medical students to school administration and, when appropriate, to the state's PHP (AMA *Code of Medical Ethics Opinion 9.3.2*; Sudan [34]). This protects public health and safety while ensuring the ill medical student receives appropriate evaluation and treatment for a potentially lethal disorder.

Identifying concerning behavior in a medical student precedes and is separate from the assessment of a medical student-patient within the context of a forensic or therapeutic relationship; it is not advisable (and potentially harmful) to serve both roles. Concerned peers or faculty should first gather and record factual observations that are cause for concern; these are required for the first step in intervening for a potentially ill medical student, often simply termed an "intervention." A helpful framework for intervening for a medical student with behavior concerning for impairment is Knight's FRAMER acronym mnemonic, which includes fact-gathering of specific observed behaviors leading to concern, determining mandated responsibility for reporting suspected impairment, including representatives from the state PHP and medical school, beginning with a complete matter-of-fact list of the facts, and ensuring the outcome of the intervention is a comprehensive independent evaluation with clear expectations of how the results will be reported back [9, 26]. An intervention should typically be done in concert with school administration, mental health staff, and/or the state PHP [35]. The goal of this intervention is mutual agreement to immediate leave from medical school with urgent evaluation and treatment of the underlying etiology of the documented impairment in functioning. Often the underlying cause of impairment is not fully known at the time of the intervention.

Treatment

The impaired medical student with an SUD must suspend coursework and clinical responsibilities during acute treatment. This preserves the medical safety of patients whose care is impacted by the medical student and removes the medical student-patient from a healthcare environment with access to controlled substances. The treatment frame includes significant contingency management around motivation to return to school and clinical practice and permits the intensive level of care required for standard-of-care treatment. Further, the impaired medical students' treatment team is protected from untoward legal risk and distressing counter-transferential experiences of treating a patient who is placing others at risk.

A partial hospital or residential program with capacity for initial medical detoxification, including management of withdrawal syndromes, is typically the acute treatment setting. Length of stay for medical professionals is typically ~3 months of intensive care with individual and group psychotherapy, process groups, family therapy, recreational therapy, a psychoeducational program targeting addiction, and introduction to the 12-step program philosophy [31, 35]. After acute stabilization, care is transferred to bi-weekly outpatient care for 3–12 months, then to ongoing care management (via the PHP) with frequent random toxicological screening, participation in community recovery support groups (e.g., Caduceus,

Alcoholics/Narcotics Anonymous, Self-Management and Recovery Training, or SMART groups), and monitoring of professional functioning through workplace monitors [11, 35].

The long-term treatment goal for medical students' and physicians' acute recovery from SUD is sustained abstinence [16, 35]. Given the chronic relapsing course of SUD, this is an ambitious but necessary outcome. Participation is motivated by the primary contingency of reporting to medical school administrators and/or state licensing authorities (and potential loss of medical licensure in the future) [35].

Medication-assisted treatment for opioid use disorder is complicated in the medical student and physician population. Treatment with opioid-receptor agonists, considered standard of care for opioid use disorder in the general population, is controversial due to concern for potential cognitive and motor impairment. Outcomes from PHPs utilizing abstinence-based treatment show that physicians with opioid use disorder have similar outcomes to physicians with alcohol- or non-opioid SUD over 5 years of intensive follow-up, suggesting that opioid-receptor agonist therapy may not be required in the physician population treated in PHPs [31]. However, a patient with multiple opioid relapses despite compliance with intensive abstinence-based treatment may indicate a need for opioid-receptor agonist or antagonist therapy [30, 35]. Naltrexone may be preferred in medical students and physicians with opioid use disorder. However, medical students and physicians with comorbid chronic pain syndromes will often require methadone or buprenorphine treatment to manage both conditions.

Psychopharmacological management of alcohol use disorder is less controversial. Four medications are approved by the US Food and Drug Administration. Daily directly observed dosing of disulfiram may be helpful in patients with engaged social supports and high levels of internal motivation for abstinence. Oral or monthly long-acting injectable naltrexone is also effective in prolonging time to relapse and reducing severity of relapses. Acamprosate may also be effective in reducing craving or "anti-reward" systems mediating relief-seeking behavior via alcohol use. Additionally, topira-mate and gabapentin have empirical evidence for efficacy in alcohol use disorder, though these are not FDA-approved and are associated with adverse cognitive effects that must be carefully weighed in the medical student population [38].

Positive outcomes are common, and sustained remission with return to clinical practice occurs in 70–80% of physicians enrolled by PHPs over 5-year follow-up [16,29,39]. Outcomes are less positive in populations without access to PHPs; only 32% of Australian-New Zealander anesthesiologists success-fully returned to work following largely outpatient-based short-duration treatment [19]. The extraordinarily high suc-cess rate with PHP-based case management is a cause for optimism in treating the medical student population and sug-gests that this level of care should be strongly considered for the medical student population.

Despite the hopeful prognosis and available evidence-based treatment, significant stigma toward addiction compli-cates the care of medical students with SUD. Physician's attitudes toward individuals diagnosed with SUDs are worse than their attitudes toward individuals with other medical and mental health diagnoses [1–4, 21, 23, 28]. Patients with addictive disorders are commonly viewed as poorly moti-vated, manipulative, and of lower importance than other patients and believed to be dangerous or violent [7, 13]. For the medical student population, the risk of misattributing SUD-related behavior to moral failing or anti-social traits is enhanced by competing needs to safeguard professional stan-dards and protect public safety. It is especially important to acknowledge and guard against the risk that stigma poses to medical students struggling with SUDs—prompt identifica-tion, referral to confidential treatment, and access to evidence-based modalities must be provided for individuals struggling with this potentially lethal disorder.

Preventive measures against the development of SUD are based largely on an epidemiological understanding of risk fac-tors. Ensuring medical students are able to attend to personal physical and mental health is of paramount importance and may curtail self-treatment of untreated disorders, as well. Regular healthcare appointments, adequate exercise, participation in self-directed leisure activities, and engagement in non-medical social activities should all be promoted by medical schools [9].

Conclusion

Rates of substance misuse and SUDs are high in medical students. Early intervention and engagement with treatment is important, and outcomes are usually positive.

References

1. Avery J, Zerbo E. Improving psychiatry residents' attitudes toward individuals diagnosed with substance use disorders. Harv Rev Psychiatry. 2015;23(4):296–300.
2. Avery J, Dixon L, Adler D, et al. Psychiatrists' attitudes toward individuals with substance use disorders and serious mental illness. J Dual Diagn. 2013;9(4):322–6.
3. Avery J, Zerbo E, Ross S. Improving psychiatrists' attitudes towards individuals with psychotic disorders and co-occurring substance use disorders. Acad Psychiatry. 2016;40(3):520–2.
4. Avery J, Han BH, Zerbo E, et al. Changes in psychiatry residents' attitudes towards individuals with substance use disorders over the course of residency training. Am J Addict. 2017;26(1):75–9.
5. Ayala EE, Roseman D, Winseman JS, Mason HRC. Prevalence, perceptions, and consequences of substance use in medical students. Med Educ Online. 2017;22:1.
6. Baldwin DC Jr, Hughes PH, Conard SE, et al. Substance use among senior medical students. A survey of 23 medical schools. JAMA. 1991;265:2074–8.
7. Ballon BC, Skinner W. "Attitude is a little thing that makes a big difference": reflection techniques for addiction psychiatry training. Acad Psychiatry. 2008;32(3):218–24.
8. Bohigian GM, Croughan JL, Sanders K, Evans ML, Bondurant R, Platt C. Substance abuse and dependence in physicians: the Missouri Physicians' Health Program. South Med J. 1996;89(11):1078–80.

9. Boyd JW, Knight JR. Substance use disorders among physicians. In: Galanter M, Kleber HD, Brady KT, editors. The American Psychiatric Publishing textbook of substance abuse treatment. 5th ed: American Psychiatric Publishing; 2015. https://psychiatryonline.org/doi/full/10.1176/appi.books.9781615370030.mg46. Accessed 1 Nov 2017.

10. Braquehais MD, Lusilla P, Bel MJ, et al. Dual diagnosis among physicians: a clinical perspective. J Dual Diagn. 2014;10(3):148–55.

11. Braquehais MD, Tresidder A, DuPont RL. Service provision to physicians with mental health and addiction problems. Curr Opin Psychiatry. 2015;28:324–9.

12. Brooke D, Edwards G, Taylor C. Addiction as an occupational hazard: 144 doctors with drug and alcohol problems. Addiction. 1991;86(8):1011–6.

13. Capurso NA, Shorter DI. Changing attitudes in graduate medical education: a commentary on attitudes towards substance use and schizophrenia by Avery et al. Am J Addict. 2017;26(1):83–6.

14. Choi D, Tolova V, Socha E, Samenow CP. Substance use and attitudes on professional conduct among medical students: a single-institution study. Acad Psychiatry. 2013;37(3):191–5.

15. Clark DC, Daugherty SR. A norm-referenced longitudinal study of medical student drinking patterns. J Subst Abus. 1990;2: 15–37.

16. Earley PH. Physician health programs and addiction among physicians. In: Ries RK, Fiellin DA, Miller SC, Saitz R, editors. The ASAM principles of addiction medicine. 5th ed. New York: Wolters Kluwer; 2014.

17. Flaherty JA, Richman JA. Substance use and addiction among medical students, residents, and physicians. Psychiatr Clin North Am. 1993;16(1):189–97.

18. Frank E, Elon L, Naimi T, et al. Alcohol consumption and alcohol counselling behaviour among U.S. medical students: cohort study. BMJ. 2008;337:a2155.

19. Fry RA, Fry LE, Castanelli DJ. A retrospective survey of substance abuse in anesthetists in Australia and New Zealand from 2004 to 2013. Anaesth Intensive Care. 2015;43(1):111–7.

20. Galanter M, Dermatis H, Mansch P, et al. Substance-abusing physicians: monitoring and twelve-step-based treatment. Am J Addict. 2007;16:117–23.

21. Geller G, Levine DM, Mamon JA, et al. Knowledge, attitudes, and reported practices of medical students and house staff

regarding the diagnosis and treatment of alcoholism. JAMA. 1989;262(21):3115–20.

22. Gignon M, Havet E, Ammirati C, et al. Alcohol, cigarette, and illegal substance consumption among medical students: a cross-sectional survey. Workplace Health Saf. 2015;63(2):54–63.

23. Gilchrist G, Moskalewicz J, Slezakova S, et al. Staff regard towards working with substance users: a European multi-centre study. Addiction. 2011;106:1114–25.

24. Hughes PH, Conard SE, Baldwin DC Jr, et al. Resident physician substance use in the United States. JAMA. 1991;265(16):2069–73.

25. Jackson ER, Shanafelt TD, Hasan O, et al. Burnout and alcohol abuse/dependence among U.S. medical students. Acad Med. 2016;91(9):1251–6.

26. Knight JR. A 35-year-old physician with opioid dependence. JAMA. 2004;292(11):1351–7.

27. Koob GF. Neurobiology of addiction. In: Galanter M, Kleber HD, Brady KT, editors. Textbook of substance abuse treatment. 5th ed: American Psychiatric Publishing; 2015. https://psychiatryonline.org/doi/full/10.1176/appi.books.9781615370030.mg01. Accessed 15 Oct 2017.

28. Lindberg M, Vergara C, Wild-Wesley R, et al. Physicians-in-training attitudes toward caring for and working with patients with alcohol and drug abuse diagnoses. South Med J. 2006;99(1):28–35.

29. McLellan AT, Skipper GS, Campbell M, DuPont RL. Five year outcomes in a cohort study of physicians treated for substance use disorders in the United States. BMJ. 2008;337:a2038.

30. Merlo LJ, Gold MS. Prescription opioid abuse and dependence among physicians: hypotheses and treatment. Harv Rev Psychiatry. 2008;16:181–94.

31. Merlo LJ, Campbell MD, Skipper GE, et al. Outcomes for physicians with opioid dependence treated without agonist pharmacotherapy in physician health programs. J Subst Abus Treat. 2016;64:47–54.

32. Merlo LJ, Curran JS, Watson R. Gender differences in substance use and psychiatric distress among medical students: a comprehensive statewide evaluation. Subst Abus. 2017;38(4):401–6.

33. Oreskovich MR, Shanafelt T, Dyrbye LN, et al. The prevalence of substance use disorders in American physicians. Am J Addict. 2015;24:30–8.

34. Physician responsibilities to impaired colleagues. In: Code of Medical Ethics Opinion 9.3.2. American Medical Association.

2016. https://www.ama-assn.org/delivering-care/physician-responsibilities-impaired-colleagues. Accessed 1 Nov 2017.
35. Physician health program guidelines. Federation of State Physician Health Programs. Dec 2005. http://www.fsphp.org/sites/default/files/pdfs/2005_fsphp_guidelines-master_0.pdf. Accessed 30 Oct 2017.
36. Policy on physician impairment. Federation of State Medical Boards. Apr 2011. https://www.fsmb.org/Media/Default/PDF/FSMB/Advocacy/grpol_policy-on-physician-impairment.pdf. Accessed 1 Nov 2017.
37. Public policy statement: physician illness vs. impairment. Federation of State Physician Health Programs. Jul 2008. https://www.fsmb.org/Media/Default/PDF/FSMB/Advocacy/grpol_policy-on-physician-impairment.pdf. Accessed 1 Nov 2017.
38. Reus VI, Fochtmann LJ, Bukstein O, et al. The American Psychiatric Association practice guideline for the pharmacological treatment of patients with alcohol use disorder. Am J Psychiatry. 2018;175:86–90.
39. Rose JS, Campbell M, Skipper G. Prognosis for emergency physician with substance abuse recovery: 5-year outcome study. West J Emerg Med. 2014;15(1):20–5.
40. Shah AA, Bazargan-Hejazi S, Lindstrom RW, et al. Prevalence of at-risk drinking among a national sample of medical students. Subst Abus. 2009;30:141–9.
41. The sick physician: impairment by psychiatric disorders, including alcoholism and drug dependence. JAMA. 1973;223(6):684–687.
42. Weiss Roberts L, Warner TD, Rogers M, et al. Medical student illness and impairment: a vignette-based survey study involved 955 students at 9 medical schools. Compr Psychiatry. 2005;46:229–37.
43. Wile C, Frei M, Jenkins K. Doctors and medical students case managed by an Australian Doctors Health Program: characteristics and outcomes. Australas Psychiatry. 2011;19(3):202–5.
44. Yarborough WH. Substance use disorders in physician training programs. J Okla State Med Assoc. 1999;92(10):504–7.
45. Cheng J, Kumar S, Nelson E, Harris T, Coverdale J. A national survey of medical student suicides. Acad Psychiatry. 2014;38(5):542–6.

Chapter 4
Mindfulness

Chiti Parikh

Introduction to Mindfulness

The term mindfulness is ubiquitous these days in almost every field. Chances are you might have come across it on the news, medical journals, pop culture, bookstores, or even the app store. Lately more and more attention is being paid towards chronic stress and how it affects our physical, psychological, and spiritual well-being. As we see an increase in awareness on impact of stress, we also see more stress management techniques being researched and implemented across various settings. Employers such as Google, Facebook, and many more are coming up with innovative ideas to reduce stress in the work environment to improve productivity and employee satisfaction [17]. As millennials enter the workforce, they are looking for careers that offer them better work–life balance. To attract top candidates, employers are not only enticing them with salaries and bonuses but through flexible work schedules, onsite gyms, day cares, resiliency training, and more vacation days [24].

C. Parikh (✉)
Weill Cornell Medicine/New York Presbyterian Hospital/
Integrative Health and Wellbeing, New York, NY, USA

© Springer Nature Switzerland AG 2019
D. Zappetti, J. D. Avery (eds.), *Medical Student Well-Being*,
https://doi.org/10.1007/978-3-030-16558-1_4

The main theme in these changing trends is the acknowledgement of stress and its negative impact on all aspects of human experience. Words like mindfulness might be in vogue now but the human condition has been plagued with stress throughout history. Not surprisingly, most ancient cultures and traditions have looked into this issue as we are doing now. Traditions of zen, meditation, and yoga have been around for millennia, and we have a lot to learn from them.

So what is mindfulness and what is the buzz really about? It has been defined in many ways. Jon Kabat-Zinn, the creator of mindfulness-based stress reduction program, defines "Mindfulness as paying attention in a particular way: on purpose, in the present moment, and nonjudgmentally," whereas zen master Thich Nhat Hanh states that "Mindfulness shows us what is happening in our bodies, our emotions, our minds, and in the world. Through mindfulness, we avoid harming ourselves and others." If we asked all the experts in the field, each one would define it slightly differently. However, the common themes of observation, awareness, attention, and nonjudgment surface in all definitions.

The terms mindfulness and meditation are often used interchangeably. The practice of mindfulness is meditation. When we think of meditation, an image of a yogi sitting under a tree with eyes closed and chanting a secret mantra comes to mind. Most people think meditation is something to be practiced in a quiet setting, sitting down in a certain posture while focusing on an image or a mantra, all the while trying to stop your thoughts. In reality, this concept is the opposite of what mindfulness represents. One does not need to be in any particular setting or posture to be mindful. Meditation or mindfulness can be practiced anywhere, anytime, and by anyone. Just by being aware of the present moment without disappearing into the past or the future, one is meditating.

In our fast-paced lives, we constantly find ourselves "multitasking" where we might be writing an email but we are thinking about the grocery list, when you will pick up your kids, or some comment your boss made a month ago. This illusion of multitasking is just that, an illusion. Just as we cannot be physically present at multiple locations, our mind cannot juggle multiple chains of thoughts effectively. What we are really doing is jumping between different thoughts rapidly without completion. This leads to more chaos in the mind and feeling of anxiety.

Mindfulness teaches us to be present in the given moment, paying full attention to task at hand without getting distracted. Through focused attention we can accomplish any task faster, with greater efficiency and accuracy. Sounds very simple doesn't it. And it is. As easy as riding a bike. Seems like an unsurmountable task at first but once you get a hang out of it, it comes effortlessly.

Biological Effects of Stress

One of the major applications of meditation is for stress management. The physiologic response to stress is governed by our autonomic nervous system which is involuntary. It is responsible for vital functions such as regulation of respiration, heart rate, blood pressure, skin temperature, digestion, and sexual function. The autonomic nervous system has two facets, sympathetic and parasympathetic nervous system.

The sympathetic nervous system is activated during stress and is often referred to as the "fight-or-flight" response. Hormones such as cortisol and adrenaline are secreted when the sympathetic nervous system is activated. These hormones in turn increase our blood pressure, respiratory rate, and heart rate, so our body can maintain circulation. It does this by shunting blood away from the digestive tract and sex organs to muscles, heart, and brain. During acute stress this "fight-or-flight" response is vital to our survival.

Whereas the parasympathetic nervous system helps us recover from stress by activating the vagus nerve often referred to as the "rest and digest" system, it decreases our blood pressure, respiratory rate, and heart rate while increasing the blood supply to the gastrointestinal and reproductive organs.

Thousands of years ago when our ancestors were living in caves, battling severe weather conditions, starvation, and disease, they relied on their stress response for their survival during difficult times. Our body has evolved to prioritize the stress response and production of hormones such as cortisol at the expense of other physiologic functions that are not as important for survival.

However, when the sympathetic nervous system is active chronically, it starts to have a negative impact on our physiology. Chronic elevation in blood levels of cortisol and adrenaline can increase blood pressure, blood sugar, and suppress our immune system. Chronic stress has been linked to increased incidence of heart disease, hypertension, stroke, and diabetes. In our modern world, we do not have to worry about fighting the elements, starvation, or diseases like our ancestors. Our triggers for activating the "fight-or-flight" response can be something a lot less threatening such as studying for a test, running late to work, or arguing with a family member. All of these daily tasks can trigger the sympathetic nervous system multiple times a day. Most of us do not even realize that we are often stuck in this mode and grow accustomed to being chronically stressed.

Mindfulness or meditation helps us recover from the stress response by activating the parasympathetic nervous system [39]. Other activities such as praying, being in nature, laughing, expressing gratitude [23], yoga, and exercise [19] have shown to have a similar effect. Perhaps this is the reason we often feel relaxed and happy when we engage in these activities.

Neurological Impact of Meditation

To appreciate the neuromodulatory effects of mindfulness, let us discuss the two main neural networks, which are a group of anatomically distinct regions in the brain that are functionally related. These are task-positive network (TPN) and the default mode network (DMN).

These neural networks are often anticorrelated, and their activity can be visualized through fMRI studies as seen in Fig. 4.1 [12]. While focusing on a specific task, the TPN is often activated, and the DMN deactivated. Abnormal activation of the DMN during TPN activity or changes in connectivity between different areas of the DMN has been associated with psychological disorders such as anxiety [33], depression [29], autism [2], attention deficit hyperactivity disorder [35], and Alzheimer's disease [16].

The main nodes of the DMN have been identified as the medial prefrontal cortex, anterior and posterior cingulate cortices, precuneus, inferior parietal cortex, and lateral temporal cortex. Although they are anatomically separate, they are connected functionally.

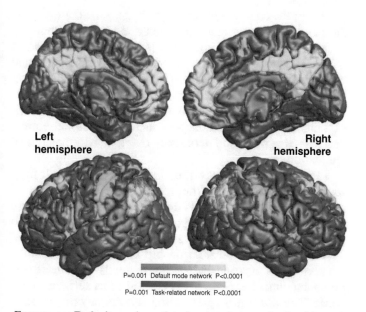

FIGURE 4.1 Default mode and task-related maps for healthy subjects. (Source: Shim et al. [30])

DMN is activated during the process of self-reflective thought, envisioning future events, mind wandering, and considering the thoughts and perspectives of others which often leads to unhappiness [4].

Whereas the TPN located mostly in the frontal and parietal regions of the brain is increasingly activated as the attention demand or the complexity of the task increases. This also leads to proportional decrease in the DMN activity [31].

Several studies have shown reduced activity of DMN during several types of meditation techniques. A recent meta-analysis found that DMN activity was consistently reduced during both focused attention and mantra-based meditation that involve repetition of phrases [34]. Similar findings were observed by Brewer et al. who compared meditators with controls across three different mindfulness meditations: focused concentration, loving kindness, and choiceless awareness.

One of the common observations by new meditators is the difficulty in focusing one's attention due to mind wandering or self-referential thinking which is related to activation of DMN. This back and forth can often lead to frustration and be one of the common reasons for discontinuation of practice. With more consistent practice, studies have shown modulation of the DMN and increase in TPN activity [31]. This explains the common findings of increased focus, attention, decrease in anxiety, and depression overtime with practice of meditation.

Vago and Silbersweig [36] have developed a framework to understand the neurobiological mechanisms of mindfulness. Mindfulness is described through systematic mental training that develops self-awareness, an ability to modulate one's behavior through self-regulation and developing a positive relationship between self and others that goes beyond self-focused needs and increases prosocial characteristics also referred to as self-transcendence. The authors suggest using this framework of self-awareness, regulation, and transcendence to inform future research in this field.

Applications of Mindfulness

There are numerous forms of meditative practices that have evolved over millennia. Some of the more common ones that have been well studied include transcendental meditation, mindfulness-based stress reduction (MBSR), loving kindness meditation (LKM), body scan meditation, and mindful breathing. Most of these types of meditations either involve open attention or focusing on breathing, mantra, visualization, or emotions.

Mindful breathing is not a formal approach, but it is commonly practiced in different settings, whether it is just taking deep breathes when one is stressed or where one will take a deep breathe, hold it for a few seconds, and exhale. The goal is to focus on the breath instead of thoughts in a nonjudgmental manner.

Another common practice is progressive muscle relaxation which is based on adaptation originally described by Edmund Jacobson. Participants start out by focusing on a slow-paced breathe, followed by focusing attention on different muscle groups in the body. Some practices ask participants to tense and then relax these muscle groups.

We will review two of the most common and well-researched practices called loving kindness meditation and mindfulness-based stress reduction.

Loving Kindness Meditation

Origins of loving kindness meditation lie in the beliefs of Theravada school of Buddhism. In this tradition, there is a concept of four different types of virtues also known as *Brahmaviharas*. Each of these virtues or mental states is associated with different meditation practices to cultivate them.

- Loving kindness (Metta)
- Compassion (Karuna)
- Empathetic joy (Mudita)
- Equanimity (Upekkha)

Each of these virtues has an opposite state that one wishes to avoid and a near opposite state which can be misunderstood as the virtue itself.

For instance, loving kindness helps one cultivate benevolence by wishing for others' happiness and well-being. The opposite state would be that of anger or resentment. Near opposite would be conditional love where one wishes well for others only if these feelings are reciprocated. The practice of loving kindness helps one wish happiness for others unconditionally, while detaching from any expectations.

The state of compassion teaches one to feel the suffering of others and wanting them to be free of it. In this case the opposite state would be inflicting suffering by being cruel, whereas the near opposite state would be of pity where one acknowledges others' suffering but does nothing to alleviate it.

Empathetic joy is rejoicing in happiness of others even if you had nothing to do with it. The opposite state would be that of jealousy and hatred toward others' happiness. The near opposite would be congratulating others on their fortune without being authentic.

Equanimity is reaching a state where you treat all beings with the highest regard irrespective of how they treat you. It is opposite of partiality or favoritism that makes you treat people differently based on how they have treated you in the past. The near opposite of this is indifference where one treats people with equal disregard.

Loving kindness meditation helps one cultivate the virtue of Metta which stands for friendship or benevolence. The concept behind this meditative practice is derived from the Metta Sutta. The following verse derived from the Metta Sutta summarizes the philosophy and practice of loving kindness meditation.

> Let none deceive another,
>   Or despise any being in any state.
> Let none through anger or ill-will
>   Wish harm upon another.
> Even as a mother protects with her life

Her child, her only child,
So with a boundless heart
Should one cherish all living beings;
Radiating kindness over the entire world:
Spreading upwards to the skies,
And downwards to the depths;
Outwards and unbounded,
Freed from hatred and ill-will.
Whether standing or walking, seated or lying down
Free from drowsiness,
One should sustain this recollection.
This is said to be the sublime abiding.
By not holding to fixed views,
The pure-hearted one, having clarity of vision,
Being freed from all sense desires,
Is not born again into this world.

"Karaniya Metta Sutta: The Buddha's Words on Loving-kindness" (Khp 9), translated from the Pali by The Amaravati Sangha.

There are four main steps in loving kindness mediation. The first step is receiving loving kindness from someone you love the most, followed by sending your loving kindness to that person. After that you send loving kindness to people you either have neutral or negative feelings for. At the end you send loving kindness to all beings in the world. One expresses loving kindness by repeating certain phrases.

Emma Seppala, Ph.D., is the Science Director, Stanford Center for Compassion and Altruism Research and Education, and has researched and written about loving kindness meditation. The following guide draws from her work.

To start your practice, sit comfortably with your feet on the ground with your eyes closed. Throughout the practice, try to keep your eyes closed and keep your attention inward. If you lose your concentration, just come back to your practice without any judgment or stress.

Receiving Loving Kindness
Think of a person in your life either in the present or in the past who has loved you unconditionally. This could be a

parent, mentor, teacher, or significant other who is currently in your life or has passed. As you think of this person, imagine they are standing on your right side and sending you their love and wishes for your happiness and well-being. Feel the warmth of their love all around you.

Now imagine another person, or the same person who loves you very much standing on your left side. Picture all of your loved ones standing around you, as they send their wishes for your happiness, health, and well-being. Now you are overflowing with their warm and unconditional love.

Sending Loving Kindness to Loved Ones

Bring your attention back to the person on your right side who you love very much, as they love you. Now send all of the warm wishes you received back to them.

You may repeat any of the following phrases silently:

> *May you live with ease, may you be happy, may you be free from pain.*
> *Just as I wish to, may you be safe, may you be healthy, may you live with ease and happiness.*
> *May your life be filled with happiness, health, and well-being.*

Now send your wishes and your love to the person on your left and so on.

Sending Loving Kindness to Neutral or Negative

Now think of an acquittance or someone you have not known for long or do not know much about them and someone you do not have any specific positive or negative feelings toward. This could be a coworker, someone you go to school with, or a neighbor. Send all of your good wishes for their well-being by repeating the following phrases silently.

> *Just as I wish to, may you also live with ease and happiness.*
> *May you be happy, may you be healthy, may you be free from all pain.*

Continue this exercise by thinking of someone you might have negative feelings toward, someone who might have hurt you in the past, or someone who has not reciprocated the feelings you have expressed for them. Send them your unconditional love and wish for their happiness and health.

Sending Loving Kindness to All Living Beings
Now spread the vastness of your love to include the whole world and all beings. Let your love fill every inch of this world. Every being wants to be happy, healthy, and free of pain just as you do.

Just as I wish to, may you live with ease, happiness, and good health.

Slowly take a deep breathe in and out as you conclude the meditation, and notice how you feel mentally, emotionally, and psychologically after the meditation. When you are ready gently open your eyes.

Physiologic Impact of Loving Kindness Meditation

Several studies have assessed the neural response to LKM. Most of the impact is on the DMN involved in self-related processing and mind wandering, an effect that is commonly seen across different meditation practices. Compared to other meditation techniques, LKM also has an effect on the emotional or affective processing [13].

Recent study conducted at Yale University aimed to assess the neural substrate of loving kindness meditation. It compared 20 meditators with over 9 years of experience with 26 novices with no prior meditation experience. All participants were asked to think of a time when they genuinely wished someone well and as they focused on this feeling silently they underwent fMRI scanning. The findings indicated that experienced meditators activate regions of the brain involved with empathy, social cognition, inner speech, and memory process. Meditators also had less activation of brain areas involved in self-related thoughts and mind wandering compared to novices. This highlights the benefit of loving kindness mediation in increasing awareness on the present moment by shifting focus away from self onto others [18].

In more experienced meditators of LKM, an increase in gray matter volume has been detected in areas of left temporal lobe and posterior parahippocampal gyri which has been observed in other forms of meditation as well. However, the changes in right angular gyrus, an area involved in affective regulation, is unique to loving kindness meditation [25]. Some of the other physiologic changes noted through LMK besides gray matter changes have been modulation of the stress response. This has been assessed by change in vagal tone or activation of the parasympathetic system, increase in telomere length, and increase in respiratory sinus arrhythmia.

Clinical Applications of Loving Kindness Meditation

How long does one have to meditate before any benefits are tangible? The benefits of LKM depend on the amount of experience of the meditator. However, some of the beneficial effects can be seen even in a single session of less than 10 minutes. Study by Hutcherson et al. [18] showed an increase in social connection and positivity toward stranger compared to closely matched controls in just one session of 10 minutes with no prior meditation experience, whereas more experienced meditators do develop noticeable gray matter changes in certain areas of the brain as seen on different imaging modalities.

What if one learns LKM and notices benefits after a few months? Would they lose all of these benefits if they stopped meditating or does some indelible impact persist?

Cohn and Fredrickson showed that some benefits of LKM persisted after 15 months even if the subjects did not continue the practice. These benefits were in the areas of social and psychological resources such as mindfulness, psychological and social well-being, hope, ego-resilience, social support, etc. The ones that did continue the practice reported more positive emotions and a more rapid positive emotion response as well [5].

LKM increases positive emotions and decreases negative emotions. It also increases compassion and social connection while decreasing self-criticism and bias toward others.

Clinical benefit of LKM has been shown in several conditions such as PTSD, depression, chronic pain, migraines, and schizophrenia. A pilot study by Kearney et al. [20] looked at measures of PTSD, depression, self-compassion, and mindfulness at a baseline, after a 12-week loving kindness meditation course and 3-month follow-up. With a 74% attendance rate, the study found reduction in PTSD symptoms and depression through enhanced self-compassion [20].

One of the key benefits of LKM is that it can be self-learned through free online resources. It does not require a minimum literacy level to follow or understand the instructions. Its benefits are comparable to other mindfulness practices without the time or resource requirements. This allows for a more cost- and time-effective implementation for any individual or institution.

Mindfulness-Based Stress Reduction

MBSR was founded by Dr. Jon Kabat-Zinn in 1979 while working at the University of Massachusetts. The course focuses on teaching mindfulness meditation and its application to overcome challenges one faces in daily life. It combines aspects of meditation, yoga, and inquiry to increase awareness of one's thoughts and reactions. It was originally developed for patients with chronic pain who had diagnosis of cancer, AIDS, and other serious illness but has since expanded its application to include stress experienced on a day-to-day basis which can sometimes be overwhelming even without a medical diagnosis.

MBSR has been the most researched formal mindfulness-based practice. Research conducted on MBSR in the last three decades has found it to be helpful with a myriad of medical and psychological conditions.

It is an 8-week intensive training course with 2.5-hour sessions every week followed by a daylong silent meditation retreat. It does require a 45–60 minute daily home meditation practice. The course is taught by an instructor who has gone through advance teacher training curriculum through University of Massachusetts. Participants are screened by the instructor since there are certain exclusion criteria for participation.

- Active substance dependence*
- Substance dependence new to recovery (less than 1 year)*
- Inadequate comprehension of language in which course is taught
- Suicidality*
- Psychosis (not treatable with medication)
- PTSD*
- Depression (clinical) or other major psychiatric diagnosis (if it interferes with participation)*
- Social anxiety (difficulty with being in a classroom situation)*
- Inability to comprehend the nature and limitations of the program
- Inability to commit to attending classes

*Some of these exclusions can be evaluated on a case-by-case basis at the discretion of the instructor and in conjunction with the participant's medical providers.

This course is suitable for individuals who are suffering from stress or its impact on other medical conditions. Participants should be willing and able to partake in a group setting, while becoming aware of often challenging thoughts, emotions, and sensations. To get the maximum benefit, participants must commit to attending all sessions and dedicate time for home practice.

Physiological Changes with MBSR

MBSR practice leads to functional and structural changes in the prefrontal cortex, cingulate cortex, insula, and hippocampus which is similar to changes seen with other meditation practices. In addition, MBSR also leads to decreased functional activity in the amygdala consistent with improved emotional regulation since increased reactivity in the amygdala is often linked to depression. Some of these changes are appreciable in just 8 weeks of MBSR training. These changes may reflect increased attentional focus, sensory processing, and reflective awareness of sensory experience [21].

One of the key applications of MBSR is in stress management. Stress induces increase in sympathetic autonomic activity which is the "fight-and-flight" response and decrease in vagal mediated parasympathetic activity which controls digestion, respiratory rate, and sexual function. Similar to other meditation techniques, MBSR leads to improvement in sympatho-vagal balance as measured by heart rate variability [28]. MBSR has also been found to reduce the amount of pro-inflammatory NH-kB-related gene expression [6].

Clinical Applications of MBSR

A systematic review of randomized controlled trials reviewed 21 articles and found that MBSR improved mental health in 11 studies compared to waitlist control or treatment as usual and was as efficacious as active control group in 3 studies [11]. It has also been found to have efficacy as adjunctive intervention for anxiety and pain management, along with benefits for general psychological health and stress management in those with medical and psychiatric illness as well as in healthy individuals [26].

Besides mood disorders, MBSR has also been effective for many other clinical conditions such as asthma, chronic pain, diabetes, gastrointestinal disorders, heart disease, and hypertension.

Comparing Different Meditation Techniques

All meditation practices tend to have a positive effect on energy, increase in focus, and decrease in the number of distracting thoughts. However, there are subtle differences between different meditation practices and these differences can be taken into account when one chooses which meditation to practice.

Kok et al. [22] found that body scan meditation where one focuses attention on different parts of the body led to the greatest state increase in interoceptive awareness and the greatest decrease in thought content, whereas loving kindness meditation led to the greatest increase in feelings of warmth and positive thoughts about others, and observing-thought meditation led to the greatest increase in metacognitive awareness [22].

Authors of the study also looked at differences in physiologic response to different meditation techniques. They noted an increase in heart rate and decrease in heart rate variability and effort over 3 months for loving kindness meditation and observing-thought meditation compared to breathing meditation. This study also highlights another important fact that certain meditation techniques such as loving kindness meditation require effort and can cause psychological arousal compared to breathing meditation which tends to require less effort.

Decentering has been another proposed mechanism for mindfulness-based practices. It emphasizes the ability to experience one's self as separate from one's thoughts and feelings and ability to observe them without analyzing or attempting to change them. When comparing mindful breathing, progressive muscle relaxation, and loving kindness meditation, MB caused more decentering, whereas among participants in PMR and LKM, there was a strong correlation between frequency of repetitive thought and negative reactions to thoughts [10].

Applications of Mindfulness in Medical School

As students enter medical school training, it earmarks the beginning of an extremely stressful time of their life. They often suffer from burnout, anxiety, and depression, a trend seen worldwide, not just in the United States. The stress management skills students develop during this time can set the tone for how they cope with stress not just as a student but also as a resident and beyond. Compared to their age-matched peers in the US general population, 50% of medical students score at least half of a standard deviation higher on perceived stress scores [8]. Given this trend, more attention is being paid to the importance of self-care and development of stress management techniques in medical school training.

A study published in BMC Medical Education assessed the impact of engagement in self-care behaviors on relationship between stress and quality of life among medical students. An online questionnaire was completed by 871 medical students across 49 medical colleges in the USA. The survey assessed self-care, perceived stress, quality of life, and demographic variables. The study showed that self-reported engagement in self-care is associated with a decrease in the relationship between perceived stress and quality of life [3].

Several medical schools have developed programs to incorporate mindfulness into the curriculum. Some of these programs include the formal MBSR training, whereas other programs include concept of mindfulness in a more informal manner. Before we review different approaches to including mindfulness into the medical school curriculum, it is important to ask if the students are genuinely interested in these interventions or are we simply adding more on their overflowing plates.

Van Dijk et al. assessed interest among 4th year medical students in MBSR training. The study found that 53% of the students expressed interest in participating in MBSR training. These interested students also scored significantly higher on psychological distress, worrying, and problem voidance and lower on mindfulness skills compared to the non-interested students [37]. By offering mindfulness in the curriculum, we can attract students who need it the most.

The timing when mindfulness should be introduced into the curriculum, preclinical vs clinical years, is up for debate. In this study the interest and participation rates in MBSR among clinical clerkship 4th year students were higher than the rates found in other studies that focused on preclinical students. As medical school curriculum goes through major overhaul, each institution will have to consider the demands of the curriculum and when it would be best to introduce mindfulness into it.

MBSR-Based Programs

Many medical schools have adapted either the full MBSR curriculum or an abridged version of it to improve stress management and resilience among medical students. Following is a summary of findings from studies done across the world on MBSR or other mindfulness-based interventions.

Erogul et al. [9] found that an abridged MBSR intervention improves perceived stress and self-compassion. Fifty-eight first year medical students participated in an 8-week MBSR intervention which consisted of 75 minutes of weekly class time, meditation at home, and a half-day retreat [9].

A Norwegian study looked at mental distress, study stress, subjective well-being, and mindfulness after participating in the MBSR program. 288 medical and psychology students participated and 76% of the participants were females. Interestingly, female medical and psychology students experienced significant positive improvement in all of the metrics compared to male students. This gender-specific response has not been noted in previous studies. The study went on to investigate the 6-year effects of the mindfulness intervention. It found that students receiving mindfulness training reported increased well-being along with increases in the trajectory of dispositional mindfulness and problem-focused coping along with greater decreases in the trajectory of avoidance-focused coping. These effects were found despite relatively low levels of adherence to formal mindfulness practice. The findings demonstrate the long-term effects and viability of mindfulness training in promotion of well-being and enhanced coping skills. MBSR course might seem like a significant investment of time and resources but one must consider its long-term benefits [38].

A study published in Canadian Medical Education Journal developed a peer-led MBSR-adapted program. The authors chose to create a peer-led program since it may be perceived as less stigmatizing than a program led by mental health professionals or medical faculty. It was an 8-week-long program specially designed for medical students by addressing issues such as work–life balance, dealing with patient suffering and perfectionism. It was led by medical students who underwent formal MBSR training. The intervention decreased levels of stress and enhanced mindfulness, self-compassion, and altruism from a baseline to post-study; however, compliance was suboptimal [7].

Greeson et al. [15] developed an adapted 4-week mind–body skills group for medical students. With 44 participants from a large southeastern US medical school, 82% completed the workshop. Students reported that the program helped them cope more skillfully with stress and increase self-care behaviors such as exercise, sleep, and engaging in social support. The authors point out that even a brief 4-week voluntary mindfulness intervention designed for medical students is feasible and effective in reducing stress, increasing mindfulness, and encouraging self-care behavior [15].

Far-Reaching Benefits of Mindfulness

Mindfulness training can benefit the students in addressing stress and improving mental health, while improving their overall education experience. A study by Xu et al. [40] looked at educational environment measure and mindfulness skills among Chinese medical students and found that higher mindfulness scores were associated with greater satisfaction with the educational environment and this association persisted a year later. The authors noted that "given that mindfulness is an inherent ability that all people can develop, medical students may benefit from instruction in mindfulness skills, especially in the areas of describing and acting with awareness, alongside the development of their professional skills" [40].

A study conducted at Monash University in Australia found a strong correlation between distress and both mindfulness and self-care. Of note, mindfulness was also a significant moderator of the relationship between several dimensions of self-care and psychological distress. Thus, mindfulness can create a foundation upon which students can develop lifelong self-care skills [32].

Making a Case for Including Mindfulness in Medical School Curriculum

A recent meta-analysis conducted by JAMA Internal Medicine reviewed 18,753 citations and included 47 trials with 3515 participants. It found that mindfulness meditation programs had moderate evidence of improved anxiety and depression at 8 weeks and 3–6 months, along with pain. It found low-level evidence of improved stress/distress and mental health-related quality of life [14].

Just as we learn lifesaving skills such as CPR to save lives of others, shouldn't we, as healthcare providers, be equipped with skills to improve our resilience and well-being? The effects of learning mindfulness are far reaching beyond the four walls of the hospital or medical school. It helps us cope with all sorts of life stressors and emerge more resilient than before.

While one is exposed to inordinate amount of stress during medical training, one can develop either constructive or destructive ways of coping with it. A 2013 study in the Journal of Addiction Medicine revealed that 69% of doctors abused prescription medicine "to relieve stress and physical or emotional pain" [27]. With greater access to prescription medicines, healthcare providers find themselves at a higher risk of dependency.

With recent rise in burnout, substance abuse, mental health conditions, and suicide rates among students, residents, and experienced physician, we need to take a closer look at the opportunity we have during the four years of medical school training to cultivate skills to better navigate what is often a highly physically, psychologically, and emotionally demanding career.

Let us equip our students with tools to "heal thyself." We can accomplish this by incorporating evidence-based, effective, and cost and time conscious mindfulness-based interventions. These programs can teach constructive ways of dealing with unavoidable stress one faces in training and throughout the medical career. Otherwise our future generation of doctors is just as susceptible if not more at risk of maladaptive behaviors that can be damaging to their psychological and physical health.

References

1. American Psychological Association. American Psychological Association, www.apa.org/helpcenter/stress-body.aspx.
2. Assaf M, et al. Abnormal functional connectivity of default mode sub-networks in autism spectrum disorder patients. NeuroImage. 2010;53(1):247–56.
3. Ayala EE, et al. U.S. medical students who engage in self-care report less stress and higher quality of life. BMC Med Educ. 2018;18(1):189.
4. Brewer JA, et al. Meditation experience is associated with differences in default mode network activity and connectivity. Proc Natl Acad Sci. 2011;108(50):20254–9.
5. Cohn MA, Fredrickson BL. In search of durable positive psychology interventions: predictors and consequences of long-term positive behavior change. J Posit Psychol. 2010;5(5):355–66.
6. Creswell JD, et al. Mindfulness-based stress reduction training reduces loneliness and pro-inflammatory gene expression in older adults: a small randomized controlled trial. Brain Behav Immun. 2012;26(7):1095–101.
7. Danilewitz M, Bradwejn J, Koszycki D. A pilot feasibility study of a peer-led mindfulness program for medical students. Can Med Educ J. 2016;7(1):e31–7.
8. Dyrbye LN, et al. Efficacy of a brief screening tool to identify medical students in distress. Acad Med. 2011;86(7):907–14.
9. Erogul M, et al. Abridged mindfulness intervention to support wellness in first-year medical students. Teach Learn Med. 2014;26(4):350–6.

10. Feldman G, et al. Differential effects of mindful breathing, progressive muscle relaxation, and loving-kindness meditation on decentering and negative reactions to repetitive thoughts. Behav Res Ther. 2010;48(10):1002–11.
11. Fjorback LO, et al. Mindfulness-based stress reduction and mindfulness-based cognitive therapy – a systematic review of randomized controlled trials. Acta Psychiatr Scand. 2011;124(2):102–19.
12. Fox MD, et al. From the cover: the human brain is intrinsically organized into dynamic, anticorrelated functional networks. Proc Natl Acad Sci. 2005;102(27):9673–8.
13. Garrison KA, et al. BOLD signal and functional connectivity associated with loving kindness meditation. Can J Chem Eng, Wiley-Blackwell, 12 Feb 2014, onlinelibrary.wiley.com/doi/10.1002/brb3.219/full.
14. Goyal M, et al. Meditation programs for psychological stress and well-being: a systematic review and meta-analysis. Deutsche Zeitschrift Für Akupunktur. 2014;(3).
15. Greeson JM, et al. An adapted, four-week mind–body skills group for medical students: reducing stress, increasing mindfulness, and enhancing self-care. Explore. 2015;11(3):186–92.
16. Greicius MD, et al. Default-mode network activity distinguishes Alzheimer's disease from healthy aging: evidence from functional MRI. Proc Natl Acad Sci. 2004;101(13):4637–42.
17. Hershatter A, Epstein M. Millennials and the world of work: an organization and management perspective. SpringerLink, Springer, 5 Mar 2010, link.springer.com/article/10.1007/s10869-010-9160-y.
18. Hutcherson CA, et al. The neural correlates of social connection. Cogn Affect Behav Neurosci. 2014;15(1):1–14.
19. Jones S Mw, et al. A yoga & exercise randomized controlled trial for vasomotor symptoms: effects on heart rate variability. Complement Ther Med. 2016;26:66–71.
20. Kearney DJ, et al. Loving-kindness meditation for posttraumatic stress disorder: a pilot study. J Trauma Stress. 2013;26(4):426–34.
21. Kilpatrick LA, et al. Impact of mindfulness-based stress reduction training on intrinsic brain connectivity. NeuroImage. 2011;56(1):290–8.
22. Kok BE, Singer T. Erratum to: phenomenological fingerprints of four meditations: differential state changes in affect, mind-

wandering, meta-cognition, and interoception before and after daily practice across 9 months of training. Mindfulness. 2016;8(1):218–31.

23. Kyeong S, et al. Effects of gratitude meditation on neural network functional connectivity and brain-heart coupling. Sci Rep. 2017;7(1):5058.

24. Landrum S. Incentive programs that motivate millennial employees. Forbes, Forbes Magazine, 3 Nov 2017. www.forbes.com/sites/sarahlandrum/2017/11/03/incentive-programs-that-motivate-millennial-employees/.

25. Leung M-K, et al. Increased gray matter volume in the right angular and posterior parahippocampal gyri in loving-kindness meditators. Soc Cogn Affect Neurosci. 2012;8(1):34–9.

26. Marchand WR. Mindfulness-based stress reduction, mindfulness-based cognitive therapy, and zen meditation for depression, anxiety, pain, and psychological distress. J Psychiatr Pract. 2012;18(4):233–52.

27. Merlo LJ, et al. Reasons for misuse of prescription medication among physicians undergoing monitoring by a physician health program. J Addict Med. 2013;7(5):349–53.

28. Nijjar PS, et al. Modulation of the autonomic nervous system assessed through heart rate variability by a mindfulness based stress reduction program. Int J Cardiol. 2014;177(2):557–9.

29. Sheline YI, et al. The default mode network and self-referential processes in depression. Proc Natl Acad Sci. 2009;106(6):1942–7.

30. Shim G, Oh JS, Jung WH, et al. Altered resting-state connectivity in subjects at ultra-high risk for psychosis: an fMRI study. Behav Brain Funct. 2010;6:58. https://doi.org/10.1186/1744-9081-6-58.

31. Simon R, Maria E. The default mode network as a biomarker for monitoring the therapeutic effects of meditation. Front Psychol. 2015;6:776.

32. Slonim J, et al. The relationships among self-care, dispositional mindfulness, and psychological distress in medical students. Med Educ Online. 2015;20(1).

33. Tao Y, et al. The structural connectivity pattern of the default mode network and its association with memory and anxiety. Front Neuroanat. 2015;9:152.

34. Tomasino B, et al. Meditation-related activations are modulated by the practices needed to obtain it and by the expertise: an ALE meta-analysis study. Front Hum Neurosci. 2013;6:346.

35. Uddin LQ, et al. Network homogeneity reveals decreased integrity of default-mode network in ADHD. J Neurosci Methods. 2008;169(1):249–54.
36. Vago DR, Silbersweig DA. Self-awareness, self-regulation, and self-transcendence (S-ART): a framework for understanding the neurobiological mechanisms of mindfulness. Front Hum Neurosci. 2012;6:296.
37. Van Dijk I, et al. Mindfulness training for medical students in their clinical clerkships: two cross-sectional studies exploring interest and participation. BMC Med Educ. 2015;15(1):302.
38. Vibe MD, et al. Mindfulness training for stress management: a randomised controlled study of medical and psychology students. BMC Med Educ. 2013;13(1):107.
39. Wu S-D, Lo P-C. Inward-attention meditation increases parasympathetic activity: a study based on heart rate variability. Biomed Res. 2008;29(5):245–50.
40. Xu X, et al. Relation of perceptions of educational environment with mindfulness among Chinese medical students: a longitudinal study. Med Educ Online. 2016;21(1).

Chapter 5
Incorporating Exercise into a Busy Life in Medical School

Kerri I. Aronson and Dana Zappetti

The benefits of physical fitness have been recognized since the beginning of humankind. In prehistoric times, a man's pursuit of fitness aligned with the need to hunt and gather food for survival. As time progressed, fitness became less of a need for obtaining sustenance and evolved as symbol for status and power [1]. In Western society today, we no longer rely on such physically demanding practices to acquire food, and one's power and influence is not necessarily representative of physical fitness. Despite this, we have not lost sight of the value of exercise and physical activity to support our health and well-being. In the 1950s, Jack LaLanne, now termed the "Godfather of the Modern Fitness Movement," was a pioneer of physical fitness, broadcasting to the public on the health benefits of exercise and opening the nation's first health and fitness club [2]. Since that time we have continued to uncover the numerous advantages to engaging in

K. I. Aronson
Pulmonary and Critical Care Medicine, New York Presbyterian Hospital/Weill Cornell Medical College, New York, NY, USA
e-mail: kia9010@nyp.org; kia9010@med.cornell.edu

D. Zappetti (✉)
Weill Cornell Medical College, New York, NY, USA
e-mail: daz9001@med.cornell.edu

© Springer Nature Switzerland AG 2019
D. Zappetti, J. D. Avery (eds.), *Medical Student Well-Being*,
https://doi.org/10.1007/978-3-030-16558-1_5

97

exercise and the twenty-first century has produced a surge of fitness experts. While many may be familiar with more "conventional" types of exercise, running, weight lifting, swimming, etc., there are numerous new "trendy" approaches to physical activity that have emerged. We have the ability to choose activities that appeal to personal interests and fit efficiently into a busy schedule.

In 2008, the US Department of Health and Human Services published the first document to contain a comprehensive guideline for physical activity on behalf of the Federal Government. This was intended to be used by health professionals and policymakers as an evidence-based resource for the types of physical activity that provide meaningful health benefits. The document describes the numerous physical health benefits that accompany physical activity for people of all ages. The newest version of the document emphasizes the mental health benefits of physical activity [3, 4]. This highlights the understanding that well-being does not just include the state of one's physical health, but is also determined by psychological, emotional, and social factors. This chapter will detail the most prominent benefits derived from exercise from a physical and mental well-being perspective, as well as the evidence behind this. In addition, we will offer some recommendations as to how to incorporate exercise into the schedule of a busy full-time medical student.

Physical activity has been defined as "any bodily movement produced by skeletal muscles that results in energy expenditure." Exercise, in turn, is viewed as a planned and structured physical activity associated with a goal or specific objective [5]. The pursuit of physical activity and exercise is regulated in part by the individual; however, there are also societal and environmental factors that play a role [6]. Society often focuses on the effects of exercise for weight loss and maintaining a "healthy" physique. From years of research, we now understand that there are other numerous other physical health benefits to exercise. First, exercise is known to have a positive effect on cardiovascular health. In addition, benefits are seen related to sleep and immune function. In fact, exercise has led to improved outcomes in many chronic illnesses. In contrast, sedentary behaviors, such as time spent watching TV, have been associated with an elevated risk of chronic diseases such as obesity and type II diabetes [7].

With weight loss the benefits extend beyond a person's desired physical appearance. Weight loss reduces the risk and severity of numerous health conditions. A well-known example is diabetes mellitus. In patients with diabetes, exercise regimens are proven to be as good, if not better than medications for patients at risk for development of diabetes [8]. Current guidelines encourage the inclusion of exercise regimens in the management of diabetes and high blood pressure. Depending on the severity of a person's disease, exercise may be prescribed in place of traditional medication management.

Physical fitness correlates positively with longevity and a reduction in all-cause mortality [9]. The cardiovascular health benefits are numerous. People who willingly choose to perform physical activities more often in their leisure time tend to have lower numbers of fatal and nonfatal cardiovascular events [10]. With respect to lipid profiles, sedentary overweight people who are prescribed exercise regimens have lower low-density lipoprotein (LDL) and higher high-density lipoprotein (HDL) cholesterol levels compared to those who are not. There is also an incremental decrease in LDL with higher intensity of exercise [11]. This is partially due to the sequela of inflammation. Inflammation has been linked to the pathology of many chronic conditions including cardiovascular disease, obesity, and cancer. Exercise can be protective against the development of these conditions by exerting protective, anti-inflammatory effects [12]. While new exercise regimens performed at high intensity may at times cause tissue damage, exercise that is performed chronically at regular intervals can reduce markers of inflammation [13, 14].

Research focused on the effects of exercise on sleep has shown positive results. Benefits are seen in both healthy subjects and those with chronic insomnia disorders. Aerobic exercise has been shown improve specifically the quality of sleep in people with and without primary insomnia disorders [15, 16]. When people are asked directly about factors that promote their ability to fall asleep and their quality of sleep, exercise is reported as the most important factor for both [17]. In addition, those with a more favorable physical fitness status have more continuous and deeper sleep than those who are more sedentary [18]. People with sleep-disordered breathing such as obstructive sleep apnea (OSA) also derive benefit. Supervised exercise training has a positive effect on reducing the severity of OSA regardless of weight loss, with additional improvements in sleep efficiency, and the subjective level of daytime sleepiness. [19] These findings of improved sleep quality have held true when the same questions were asked of the general healthy population. In 2013, the National Sleep Foundation polled Americans via the "Sleep in America poll." They found that the overwhelming majority of people who reported any level of exercise also reported a fairly good or very good overall sleep quality when compared to those who did not exercise. Those who vigorously exercised reported the highest quality of sleep. Regardless of the level of exercise, those people who performed any level of exercise perceived their sleep quality to be improved on the days that they performed this activity [20].

In addition to the physical benefits that exercise and physical activity provide, there are numerous positive effects on one's mental health and well-being. In the past few decades, there has been a large focus on research related to the benefits of exercise for persons with mood disorders such as depression and anxiety. An activity as simple as walking is found to have protective effects against development of depression. We now believe that people with depression may actually derive therapeutic benefit from physical activity [21]. As practitioners and researchers have begun to explore alternative therapies for depression, exercise has been added to the list of non-medication treatment options. Many recent clinical studies have included exercise as a treatment intervention when examining therapies for depression. The majority of these studies have shown positive results. Importantly, these results have displayed long-term benefits, with exercise contributing to lower rates of depression relapse [22, 23]. The physiologic mechanisms for underlying this phenomenon are based in the neurohormonal system, with exercise having effects on neurotransmitters known to effect pathologic mood—dopamine, noradrenaline, adrenaline, and serotonin [24, 25].

Similarly, exercise has been shown to exert positive effects on anxiety symptoms in those with generalized anxiety disorders. Both resistance training and aerobic exercise have been shown to significantly improve self-reported anxiety among people with generalized anxiety disorders [26]. Aerobic exercise regimens have been used to alleviate elevated sensitivity to anxiety symptoms as seen in people prone to panic attacks and panic disorders [27].

The benefits of exercise are not limited to those with mood disorders. Physical exercise has been shown to buffer the anxiety that is accompanied by even minor life stressors. Increased participation in physical activities is associated with improved psychologic well-being in normal healthy adults. This effect is seen in a variety of the domains of well-being. A large study in Finland found that people who exercise at least two or three times per week experience less anger, cynicism, and stress than those who exercise less frequently [28]. The effects of physical activity even permeate the workplace. Exercises, both cardiovascular and resistance training, have been shown to decrease occupational psychological stress and burnout and increase productivity [29]. In their 2017 study published in Academic Medicine, Drybye and colleagues [30] surveyed 4402 medical students and found that 62.7% followed the Centers for Disease Control (CDC) guidelines of 150 minutes of aerobic activity weekly and fewer, 38.5%, adhered to the CDC guidelines of strength training on two or more days a week. However, in their survey, burnout prevalence was lower in those who did achieve these exercise goals [31].

In addition to improvements in a person's emotional health when adopting and exercise routine, one may also witness benefits in their social life. Group exercise activities through either exercise memberships, classes, or clubs are a fantastic way to meet other peers who share similar interests. This socialization is an additional contributor to a person's well-being that compliments the other physical and mental benefits of exercise that are outlined here.

Even when it may be clear that there are numerous benefits to adding physical activity one's daily routine, most often have trouble finding the time to do so. The recommendation for obtaining substantial health benefits is to perform physical activity 150–300 minutes of moderate intensity or 75–150 minutes of vigorous-intensity aerobic physical activity per week, with incorporation of additional muscle strength training [3]. As a busy medical student, the thought of adding a half hour or more of exercise may seem daunting. In a 2017 cross-sectional survey study of medical and nursing students, only 38% of medical students reached the recommended level of exercise and cited lack of time, inconvenient gym hours, and difficulty fitting exercise into the schedule as barriers to achieving an exercise goal [32]. It is true that a student may need to take a hard look at their daily activities to find a place to substitute exercise. What time is expendable or mutable to fit in 20–30 minutes of exercise?

Ideas for Incorporating Physical Fitness into Your Schedule

Physical activity can come in many forms and when choosing, be mindful that in order to continue an activity it needs to be enjoyable and also meet your needs. Considerations are:

- Cost
- Group or lone activity
- Amenities available on your school or hospital campus
- Level of commitment

It is ok to start slowly! Commit to a 15-minute walk each day and stick to it. Soon, adding time or changing the activity level will seem like a much smaller step. Table 5.1 outlines the pros and cons or some common physical fitness activities.

TABLE 5.1 Pros/cons of typical physical fitness activities

Activity type	Pros	Cons
Walking or running	Low cost with flexibility/can do with friend(s)	Safety issues if walking/running in the dark/hard on joints
School gym	No cost/easy to work out with friends/usually long hours	Might not have activity you want/ might not want to exercise near colleagues
Local gym	Usually long hours and a myriad of activities including classes and trainers	Costly/might take time to get there if not near campus
School clubs	Fosters community and exercising with those who have similar schedules	Might not be an existing club for the activity you like/responsible for planning group activities
Using stairs at work, exclusively	Low cost/frequent small bursts of activity integrated into the day	Hard if rounding with a group or if one has knee or joint issues
Exercise apps/monthly subscriptions (HIIT, yoga, etc.)	Usually cheaper than gym memberships or live exercise classes/ can use on your own schedule and in your own space	Motivation can be difficult/may need to buy some equipment (mats/weights)
Martial arts	Often have a component of meditation and concentration that can help with stress management	Potentially expensive and off campus

(continued)

TABLE 5.1 (continued)

Activity type	Pros	Cons
Workplace well-being programs	Could be integrated into the day, depending upon timing/usually free for hospital workers/ sense of community	Might be given at times of the day that do not work with your schedule
Bike/walk/run to work	Integrates exercise into workday without extra time required	Takes planning and might be logistically difficult in cold or hot weather or if commuting distance is too long

Think of the time you are investing in exercise as an investment in your health and well-being as a student but also in the future. Prioritizing exercise while in medical school will build the foundation to continue to pursue this activity as you advance in your training and your busy life in medicine.

References

1. Dalleck LC, Kravitz L. The history of fitness: from primitive to present times, how fitness has evolved and come of age. IDEA Health Fit Source. 2002;1; https://www.ideafit.com/fitness-library/the-history-of-fitness
2. Roberts S. The business of personal training. Illustrated. Champaign: Human Kinetics; 1996.
3. 2008 Physical Activity Guidelines for Americans.
4. Physical Activity Basics | Physical Activity | CDC [Internet]. [cited 2018 Dec 4]. Available from: https://www.cdc.gov/physicalactivity/basics/index.htm
5. Caspersen CJ, Powell KE, Christenson GM. Physical activity, exercise, and physical fitness: definitions and distinctions for health-related research. Public Health Rep. 1985;100(2):126–31.
6. Teixeira PJ, Carraça EV, Markland D, Silva MN, Ryan RM. Exercise, physical activity, and self-determination theory: a systematic review. Int J Behav Nutr Phys Act. 2012;9:78.

7. Hu FB, Li TY, Colditz GA, Willett WC, Manson JE. Television watching and other sedentary behaviors in relation to risk of obesity and type 2 diabetes mellitus in women. JAMA. 2003;289(14):1785–91.

8. Knowler WC, Barrett-Connor E, Fowler SE, Hamman RF, Lachin JM, Walker EA, et al. Reduction in the incidence of type 2 diabetes with lifestyle intervention or metformin. N Engl J Med. 2002;346(6):393–403.

9. Blair SN. Physical fitness and all-cause mortality. JAMA. 1989;262(17):2395.

10. Leon AS. Leisure-time physical activity levels and risk of coronary heart disease and death. JAMA. 1987;258(17):2388.

11. Kraus WE, Houmard JA, Duscha BD, Knetzger KJ, Wharton MB, McCartney JS, et al. Effects of the amount and intensity of exercise on plasma lipoproteins. N Engl J Med. 2002;347(19): 1483–92.

12. Gleeson M, Bishop NC, Stensel DJ, Lindley MR, Mastana SS, Nimmo MA. The anti-inflammatory effects of exercise: mechanisms and implications for the prevention and treatment of disease. Nat Rev Immunol. 2011;11(9):607–15.

13. Woods JA, Wilund KR, Martin SA, Kistler BM. Exercise, inflammation and aging. Aging Dis. 2012;3(1):130–40.

14. Albert MA, Glynn RJ, Ridker PM. Effect of physical activity on serum C-reactive protein. Am J Cardiol. 2004;93(2):221–5.

15. Passos GS, Poyares D, Santana MG, de Teixeira AAS, Lira FS, Youngstedt SD, et al. Exercise improves immune function, antidepressive response, and sleep quality in patients with chronic primary insomnia. Biomed Res Int. 2014;2014:498961.

16. Wang X, Youngstedt SD. Sleep quality improved following a single session of moderate-intensity aerobic exercise in older women: results from a pilot study. J Sport Health Sci. 2014;3(4):338–42.

17. Urponen H, Vuori I, Hasan J, Partinen M. Self-evaluations of factors promoting and disturbing sleep: an epidemiological survey in Finland. Soc Sci Med. 1988;26(4):443–50.

18. Edinger JD, Morey MC, Sullivan RJ, Higginbotham MB, Marsh GR, Dailey DS, et al. Aerobic fitness, acute exercise and sleep in older men. Sleep. 1993;16(4):351–9.

19. Iftikhar IH, Kline CE, Youngstedt SD. Effects of exercise training on sleep apnea: a meta-analysis. Lung. 2014;192(1): 175–84.

20. National Sleep Foundation 101.

21. Kelly P, Williamson C, Niven AG, Hunter R, Mutrie N, Richards J. Walking on sunshine: scoping review of the evidence for walking and mental health. Br J Sports Med. 2018;52(12):800–6.
22. Craft LL, Perna FM. The benefits of exercise for the clinically depressed. Prim Care Companion J Clin Psychiatry. 2004;6(3):104–11.
23. Babyak M, Blumenthal JA, Herman S, Khatri P, Doraiswamy M, Moore K, et al. Exercise treatment for major depression: maintenance of therapeutic benefit at 10 months. Psychosom Med. 2000;62(5):633–8.
24. Chaouloff F. Physical exercise and brain monoamines: a review. Acta Physiol Scand. 1989;137(1):1–13.
25. Ovid: Effects of acute physical exercise on central serotonergic systems. [Internet]. [cited 2018 Dec 13]. Available from: https://ovidsp.tx.ovid.com/sp-3.32.0a/ovidweb.cgi?QS2=434
f4e1a73d37e8c54ea12160ae198c509a416769a5617409ef701b-
be7049c9973203404dd5319dcedee409dfd2f63e1128a459f827
566dd2d466997852023bef25aef07356db399698d26179aa2b-
f9022ee9f4d08603981d1f165ac58c0f9c6f92c48ddb6f1b8a7c-
cba9cca97625f42a89b2d3abe55e38530c5366d4a08ac-
c9087684e882204ed915b3e87863c45fa13f86abc53f6669e-
c3a2ab5f2f28e35e8fd453054a8af96ce3415a9e99ae3de2060094
a28246bdb7107e7efba0334c79e84cbc78bc0de4eca645299d0a-
5b7eb899554b98e54cff90df0cb0ee586009d3fe135ddeae4aeb-
8b70e84efd414ab69658a75f81443a172b82afcabd995d1a55f-
cb82804bb2599a5d65b77a83f7bc1939af2b8e0922c5398371f6f5
6df87373612618fc935be9b3c775bf206e48d227cda619a29578ce0b
9b606ccc363e6b17fc
26. Asmundson GJG, Fetzner MG, Deboer LB, Powers MB, Otto MW, Smits JAJ. Let's get physical: a contemporary review of the anxiolytic effects of exercise for anxiety and its disorders. Depress Anxiety. 2013;30(4):362–73.
27. Evaluation of a brief aerobic exercise intervention for high anxiety sensit...: EBSCOhost [Internet]. [cited 2018 Dec 13]. Available from: http://web.b.ebscohost.com/ehost/pdfviewer/pdfviewer?vid=1&sid=46a49679-5eb6-4b48-8ae3-b93aa6693ebb%40sessionmgr103.
28. Hassmén P, Koivula N, Uutela A. Physical exercise and psychological well-being: a population study in Finland. Prev Med. 2000;30(1):17–25.

29. Bretland RJ, Thorsteinsson EB. Reducing workplace burnout: the relative benefits of cardiovascular and resistance exercise. PeerJ. 2015;9(3):e891.
30. Dyrbye LN, Satele D, Shanafelt TD. Healthy exercise habits are associated with lower risk of burnout and higher quality of life among U.S. medical students. Acad Med. 2017;92(7):1006–11.
31. Centers for Disease Control and Prevention. Physical activity for everyone. www.cdc.gov/physicalactivity/everyone/guidelines/adults.html. Accessed 1/7/19.
32. Blake H, Stanulewicz N, McGill F. Predictors of physical activity and barriers to exercise in nursing and medical students. J Adv Nurs. 2017;73(4):917–29.

Chapter 6
Religion and Spirituality Among Medical Students

Paulette Posner, Muhammad Ali, and Stephen Douglas

Introduction

The terms religion and spirituality can be hard to pin down. For some, the two terms may be practically synonymous; for others, they may feel mutually exclusive. How we think about religion and spirituality is defined within community, and yet also very personal. In the twentieth century, the tendency in the west had been to see religion and spirituality as occupying a separate set of concerns, as asking different questions, than medicine, and the ancient ties between the two disciplines are often forgotten [22]. In recent decades, however, there has been a growing scientific interest in the influence of religious and spiritual factors on healthcare outcomes, and evidence suggests that effective spiritual religious care results in better patient outcomes, including higher reported quality of life, higher satisfaction with care, and lower costs at the end of life [23]. From movements in patient-centered care, to initiatives in integrative

P. Posner · M. Ali · S. Douglas (✉)
Pastoral Care and Education Department, New York Presbyterian Hospital/Weill Cornell Medical Center, New York, NY, USA
e-mail: pap9101@nyp.org; mua9010@nyp.org; sed9075@nyp.org

© Springer Nature Switzerland AG 2019
D. Zappetti, J. D. Avery (eds.), *Medical Student Well-Being*,
https://doi.org/10.1007/978-3-030-16558-1_6

and holistic health, spirituality in healthcare has become a common topic of discussion and study. Because each clinician will inevitably interact with the spiritual lives of her patients, often at some of the most vulnerable moments in their lives, it is important for clinicians to be comfortable and competent discussing and assessing patients' spiritual needs and resources. It is also important that the clinician be aware of her own convictions and sources of connection and strength, whether or not she considers herself religious or spiritual. In the midst of the stressors of medical education, one's own sense of "what is spiritual," or "what really matters," can be an asset in her work with patients and potentially a bulwark against some of the negative effects associated with medical education, including burnout, moral distress, and compassion fatigue. In this chapter, we will discuss how religion and spirituality are defined in the healthcare context, the positive and problematic ways religion and spirituality intersect with patient care, ways in which medical school administrators can foster positive spiritual/religious coping, and, finally, how medical students can bring their own sense of spirituality and/or religion into their work in appropriate and sensitive ways, as they grow into ever more resilient, compassionate, and culturally competent learners and clinicians.

Defining Religion and Spirituality in Healthcare

There are no consensus definitions for religion or spirituality in medical literature, and it is worth noting at the outset that religion and spirituality are topics that bring with them many associations, past experiences, and strong feelings, for both patients and providers. While we might personally define each term in our own way, the field appears to be moving toward consensus in how the terms are used, and these common themes can serve as a starting point for our discussion.

Religion is often defined as set of beliefs, practices, and/or rituals that is related in some respect to a connection between humanity and the transcendent [8]. Religions vary widely, but they often involve a sense of the mystical or supernatural, and often carry a set of beliefs about what happens after death. They frequently carry codes of conduct for adherents as well as traditions, rituals, practices, beliefs, and behaviors that unify or demarcate a community [10].

The word spirituality is taken from the Latin root *spiritus*, meaning breath of life. The term historically has been associated with religion [8]; contemporary usage, however, may exist within or without—perhaps even in opposition to—a religious framework. Spirituality, as used in the healthcare context, refers most commonly to "that which gives people meaning and purpose in life" [18], and is often spoken of in terms of connection to oneself, others, the natural world, or the transcendent [15].

Medical literature in recent decades has tended to define religion as a subset of spirituality, though some cultures and individuals may make no distinction between the two terms. One's spirituality may or may not be religious, and may or may not be related to a sense of the divine. By this definition, one could have a wholly material spirituality. One might echo Antoine de Saint-Exupery's *The Little Prince* and say what is most important to her cannot be seen with the eyes, which is a spiritual perspective. Another person might very well say that her spirituality lies precisely in what is visible. The natural world, empiricism, and philosophical materialism, these are each capable of inspiring awe, giving purpose, and connecting one to others. Both religion and spirituality are multidimensional and intersectional (Fig. 6.1), and deal "with the ultimate concerns of people and [provide] personal as well as social identity within the context of a cosmic or metaphysical background" [8]. One's spirituality may include many foci that intersect and change over time. When the authors of this chapter in their work as hospital chaplains ask a patient where she finds her sense of the "spiritual," we might hear something

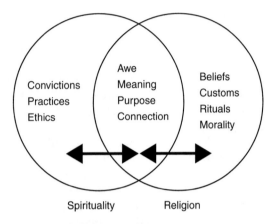

Spirituality   Religion

FIGURE 6.1 The intersection of spirituality and religion

like, "My family, my faith community, Wednesday night yoga at the community center, screen printing, activism, and my cat." Ten years later, maybe 10 minutes later, the same person might answer differently.

Spiritual Care Generalists: Culturally Competent Providers

Prayer is the most common alternative therapy in the United States, and patients frequently report wanting their doctors to address their spirituality/religion and its impact on the their medical care [3, 4]. Spiritual/religious care provided by the healthcare team has been shown to improve patient satisfaction ratings [24], create stronger patient-provider relationships [18], lower costs—particularly at the end of life [18]—and increase patient and family satisfaction with end-of-life decisions [25, 26]. Because spirituality as we have defined it is inextricable from one's culture and beliefs about life, illness, and death, spirituality and/or religion are inextricably linked to how a patient thinks, and makes decisions, about illness and health, treatment and wellness, and death and recovery, in ways that can both help and hinder coping and healing.

Despite patient preference, and despite the positive outcomes associated with spiritual/religious care provided by the healthcare team, physicians rarely report discussing these topics with patients [4], and in one study less than half of the US primary care residents felt that they should engage in spiritual care of their patients [12]. Clinicians list lack of training in spiritual and religious care as the primary barrier to discussing religion and spirituality with patients [18]. This trend may be changing. As of 2009, 85% of medical and osteopathic schools reported offering courses on spiritual care [15].

Much of the medical literature on religion and spirituality has focused on the patient's spirituality, and most commonly instances in which the patient's religious or spiritual perspective was perceived to conflict with medical ethics or the team's plan of care [7, 11, 27]. However, religion and spirituality can also be assets, not just for patients, but also for the clinicians who treat them. In recent years, a growing body of research examines how religion and spirituality influence the care clinicians provide, as well as how they cope with the stressors of their work.

In a 2018 survey of medical students, Callie Ray and Tasha Wyatt et al. point to four overarching themes among respondents: "Religion/spirituality are used as a (a) coping mechanism for the stress of medical school, (b) sense-making tool for processing difficult moments, (c) framework for making clinical/ethical decisions and for processing death, and (d) way to think about practicing patient-centered care" [17]. As chaplains at an academic medical center, we frequently hear similar themes in our conversations with medical students and residents. In an informal survey by the authors of this chapter of medical residents, many respondents endorsed that their own faith and spirituality influence and inform how they relate to patients and family, especially during end-of-life conversations. Many respondents talked about how understanding the spiritual needs of the patients could help provide what one resident called "whole-person care."

A critical tenant of the concept of whole-person care is that *healing* is distinct from *cure*. According to the World Health Organization's definition of "whole health," *cure* is focused on a disease process, whereas *healing* refers to the whole person and to how that person finds peace, a sense of coherence, solace, and/or meaning especially when dealing with loss and illness [15]. Anecdotal evidence suggests that healing is facilitated in the presence of a compassionate clinician, and in the context of that relationship [28].

In 2009, the US National Palliative Care Consensus conference met to discuss guidelines for responsible and compassionate spiritual care in the healthcare setting. The resultant document notes the "critical role" spirituality plays in the patient-provider relationship, in which "professionals and patients enter into a professional relationship whereby each party is potentially changed. Healing, as opposed to cure, is aided by the character of the provider-patient relationship" [16]. To be open to this potential change requires an awareness of the spiritual dimensions of the provider's own life and a reflective process (Ibid). Christina Puchalski et al. continue: "Many physicians and nurses speak of their own spiritual practices and how those practices help them deliver good spiritual care, which, in turn, helps in their ability to deliver good physical and psychosocial care to the seriously ill and dying patients" (Ibid). The conference guidelines name the need for reflective work, stating, "By being attentive to one's own spirituality and especially to one's sense of call to service to others, the health care professional may be able to find more meaning in his or her work and hence cope better with the stresses" (Ibid). This conception of whole-person care is a process of action and reflection in which compassionate care for the patient is linked to the clinician's own sense of meaning and care for herself.

A provider's own religion and/or spirituality can also affect the care they provide in potentially adverse ways. Research has shown that physicians' and medical students' religious beliefs influence their attitudes and decision-making around topics including death, discontinuation of life support, and abortion [1, 6, 14]. Physicians' personal religiosity has been shown to affect how they inform patients about available medical options, and how much weight they give to patients' expressed wishes in their plan of care [7, 11]. Cultural or ethical differences between providers and patients can result in considerable distress for patients, families, and providers [9]. Finally, due to as the power imbalances between the patient and clinician, there are serious ethical considerations any time a healthcare provider interacts with a patient's religion/spirituality, making it extremely important that the physician maintains personal and professional boundaries and avoids any forms of proselytizing [15].

One increasingly common way of conceiving of the physician's role in the spiritual/religious care of her patients is in terms of spiritual care specialists and generalists. In this model, a "spiritual care generalist" is any member of the healthcare team who has learned to screen for and attend to "spiritual strengths and spiritual distress and incorporate basic spiritual resources into the patient care plan" [18]. The generalist also assesses when to refer to "spiritual care specialists," such as hospital chaplains and community spiritual and religious authorities.

One of the most common and well-researched tools for spiritual assessment is known as FICA, developed by Christina Puchalski, which records a patient's *F*aith/Beliefs, *I*mportance of beliefs, her *C*ommunity, and how the patient wishes these topics to be *A*ddressed in their care [29].

This assessment may be carried out in full by a spiritual care generalist, such as a physician. In other cases, a physician may begin the assessment and then refer to a specialist. The assessment need not move linearly through these questions. It might begin with a question like, "Who are your core people?" or "What is giving you strength right now?" Regardless, the tool can serve as a guide to approaching a patient's story, including spiritual strengths and resources, as well as factors inhibiting coping.

Spirituality and Religion Among Medical Students

Medical education is famously demanding, and a growing body of research has focused on its impact on student well-being, resilience, compassion, and empathy. A 2016 review of the literature by Lauren Wasson et al. found that although matriculating US medical students begin training with significantly lower rates of depression and burnout and report better mental and emotional quality of life than other college-educated young adults, "their reported well-being decreases during the UME years" [21]. Medical students report higher rates of depression and the symptoms of burnout than other graduate students (Ibid). This decline in well-being, according to the study's authors, requires "urgent attention" (Ibid).

Medical education can often lead to students feeling isolated from the communities from which they come. "Well before entering medical school, students learn that their training will involve constant pressure and continuing fatigue. Popular stories prepare them for social isolation, the impossibility of learning everything, long hours, test anxiety, and the fact that medical school will permeate their lives" [20]. These factors "legitimate the special status of the profession the students are entering. They also blunt the students' emotional responses" [20]. In a literature review, Linda Barnes et al. conclude that "distress seems to be a main cause of empathy decline [3]." A variety of factors can lead to distress and comprise what has been referred to as a "hidden curriculum" [2]. These factors include student vulnerability, problems related to lack of social support, high workload, exhaustion, isolation, and difficult clinical realities that may not match the students' idealistic views of medicine before matriculation [2, 13].

If spirituality/religion is about connection, then it can be one tool to combat isolation—from one's family, from one's community, and from one's sense of self before embarking upon medical education—a way to return to one's roots

(Box 6.1). For students who belong to a faith tradition, student organizations such as Christian Fellowships, Muslim Students Organizations, Jewish Student Organizations, Catholic Medical Student Associations, Seventh-Day Adventist Student Organizations, and Orthodox Christian Clubs offer community—a place to celebrate holidays, share meals, and discuss medical ethics through the lens of religion. These clubs provide a wide variety of activities ranging from Bible Study, to Shabbat dinners, to weekly services and medical missions to underserved communities. Students at some schools have founded spirituality groups, open to students from any tradition or perspective, as a place to discuss their experiences and practice mindfulness, yoga, and other activities oriented toward wellness, contemplation, and resilience.

Box 6.1 Maintaining and Cultivating Connections During Medical Training

Hospitalization and illness can cut one off from the habits, activities, and people she is used to. Worse, they can separate one from how she sees herself, and how she sees herself as seen by the people in her life. The people who train and work in healthcare are also at an increased risk of feeling disconnected from their sense of self. Hospital chaplains sometimes think of their role as helping patients connect to who they are "outside" of the hospital or their illness—the activities, people, habits of mind and spirit, and practices that have brought them strength, peace, and connection throughout their lives. This might be a good way to think about your own wellness in the course of medical education. What are the things that connect you to the "You" outside of the hospital, and how can you be intentional about maintaining them throughout the hard work of medical school?

Instructors are integrating practices such as narrative medicine (see Charon et al. [5]) and "existential Fridays" (see Shand [19]) as opportunities in the classroom for students to process the emotional impact of their clinical experiences. Clubs for creative outlets such as drama, music, and art can foster growth and serve as a link to the passions, sources of inspiration, and respite that students have found meaningful in the past. At the hospital where the authors of this chapter work, medical students have the option of rotating in a clerkship program in which students shadow hospital chaplains, in which the students are invited to reflect on their own emotional/spiritual/religious responses to clinical interactions.

Religion and spirituality can function as a cultural asset for medical students and medical schools, both in the students' clinical work and as a coping resource. Respondents in one study named practices such as prayer and meditation as "an additional support system" and "an extra line of defense against the things that have become stressful or induce anxiety" [17]. Evidence suggests the benefits of spiritual care training are twofold: positive patient outcomes and more resilient providers. For instance, spiritual care training has been shown to directly benefit palliative care providers. "In one study, the clinician's spiritual well-being, compassion for oneself, and satisfaction with work increased, and work-related stress decreased following spiritual care training" [18]. Callie Ray and Tasha Wyatt et al. note "an increase in well-being when medical students focus on their spirituality" [17]. They recommend that medical schools provide opportunities for students to employ and recognize religion/spirituality as an asset, including identifying and thinking through "their own coping strategies with death," as a resource in processing the death of their patients (Ibid). Spiritual care training for medical students can be employed as part of an overall curriculum designed to increase cultural competency, and to combat empathy decline during clinical rotations [4, 13]. Melanie Neumann et al. propose the incorporation of "well-researched spiritual modalities, such as mindfulness-based stress reduction and self-awareness training, allowing students and residents to reflect on issues of vulnerability and responsibility" in healthcare [13]. The aim is to help students to reflect on their own emotional processes and to meet their patients, and themselves, with curiosity, cultural humility, and compassion.

Modalities and Personal Practices

The following are examples of spiritual practices that may be meaningful for medical students as they think about ways to incorporate what is most important to them as an asset in their work with patients and their own coping.

Creativity as Spiritual Practice

Take time to do what you love, to be creative, or quiet, or to spend time in a favorite place, even—maybe especially—when you get busy. Some examples include:

- Spend time in nature
- Take a long walk
- Talk to a friend
- Do something creative
- Cook a nice meal and eat it slowly
- Write in a journal

One exercise is to write whatever comes to your mind for 10 minutes. It might be about school or a clinical experience. It might not. The key is to keep writing without stopping. Let the critical, editing part of your mind take a break. What you write does not have to be "good." If your mind goes blank, that is okay—just write, "something will come" until something new pops into your head. When you are done, read it over and see if anything new or surprising jumps out to you.

Gratitude as Spiritual Practice

Practicing gratitude, intentionally pausing to think about the things you are thankful for, is one of the most well-researched means of combating burnout and compassion fatigue.

An example of a brief gratitude meditation: In a quiet space, allow for silence. Slowly go back over your day, from waking and getting ready until this moment. Think of the things you are grateful for, small or big. It might help to write them down. It might help to say them aloud.

Mindfulness as Spiritual Practice

There are many ways to practice mindfulness. Meditation, prayer, drawing, and physical activity are all potential ways to practice mindfulness. See the chapter on mindfulness for more ideas.

Grieving and Letting Go

Allow yourself to grieve losses fully. Allow yourself, when ready, to move on.

Conclusion

It is an exciting moment in healthcare. Just as scientific advancement opens up new therapies, modalities, and hopes for healing, so too do advancements in how hospitals and providers attend to their patients' humanity in all their diversity and particularity. To become such a provider, it is important to care for oneself. The FICA assessment tool described above can be a good way for the student or provider to check in with herself. One could ask, "What are my beliefs (*F*aith) that this case touches in me? In what way are these beliefs *I*mportant for me in this instance?

What is my Community that I can turn to now if I need to? How can I Address my own needs right now, and who can help?" Attending to these kinds of questions and answers can help us know when to return to our sources of inner strength, as well as when to reach out to trusted friends or family, or professional support.

When we in our work as chaplains ask our patients if they have a spiritual or religious practice, it is a reminder that many spiritualities and/or religions are *practices*, something we do, and are, and something that shapes us, without ever "arriving" or finishing, at least on this side of death. So too is the practice of providing care, as the clinician (or future clinician) works to attend better to the emotional/existential/spiritual/religious dimensions of her patients and herself. Medical students have certainly heard many times what a privilege, and what a challenge, medical education is by the time they begin. Our wish for you is that as you grow in knowledge and clinical acumen, the same things that brought you to this point continue to sustain you, that you discover sources of rest and inspiration throughout your career, and that you attend to your whole self with the same compassion with which you attend to those placed in your care.

References

1. Aiyer AN, Ruiz G, Steinman A, Ho GY. Influence of physician attitudes on willingness to perform abortion. Obstet Gynecol. 1999;93:576–80.
2. Balboni MJ, Bandini J, Mitchell C, Epstein-Peterson ZD, Amobi A, Cahill J, Enzinger AC, Peteet J, Balboni T. Religion, spirituality, and the hidden curriculum: medical student and faculty reflections. J Pain Symptom Manag. 2015;50:507–15.
3. Barnes LL, Plotnikoff GA, Fox K, Pendleton S. Spirituality, religion, and pediatrics: intersecting worlds of healing. Pedatrics. 2000;106:899–908.

4. Best M, Butow P, Olver I. Why do we find it so hard to discuss spirituality? A qualitative exploration of attitudinal barriers. J Clin Med. 2016;5:77.
5. Charon R, Trautmann Banks J, Connelly JE, et al. Literature and medicine: contributions to clinical practice. Ann Intern Med. 1995;122:599–606.
6. Christakis NA, Asch DA. Physician characteristics associated with decisions to withdraw life support. Am J Public Health. 1995;85:367–72.
7. Curlin FA, Lawrence RE, Chin MH, Lantos JD. Religion, conscience, and controversial clinical practices. N Engl J Med. 2007;356:593–600.
8. Hill PC, Pargament KI, Hood RW, McCullough J Michael E, Swyers JP, Larson DB, Zinnbauer BJ. Conceptualizing religion and spirituality: points of commonality, points of departure. J Theory Soc Behav. 2000;30:51–77.
9. Johnstone M-J, Kanitsaki O. Ethics and advance care planning in a culturally diverse society. J Transcult Nurs. 2009;20:405–16.
10. Koenig HG. Religion, spirituality, and health: the research and clinical implications. Int Sch Res Notices. 2012; https://doi.org/10.5402/2012/278730.
11. Lawrence RE, Curlin FA. Autonomy, religion and clinical decisions: findings from a national physician survey. J Med Ethics. 2009;35:214–8.
12. Luckhaupt SE, Yi MS, Mueller CV, Mrus JM, Peterman AH, Puchalski CM, Tsevat J. Beliefs of primary care residents regarding spirituality and religion in clinical encounters with patients: a study at a midwestern U.S. teaching institution. Acad Med. 2005;80:560–70.
13. Neumann M, Edelhäuser F, Tauschel D, Fischer MR, Wirtz M, Woopen C, Haramati A, Scheffer C. Empathy decline and its reasons: a systematic review of studies with medical students and residents. Acad Med. 2011;86:996–1009.
14. Pomfret S, Mufti S, Seale C. Medical students and end-of-life decisions: the influence of religion. Future Hosp J. 2018;5:25–9.
15. Puchalski C, Ferrell B, Virani R, et al. Improving the quality of spiritual care as a dimension of palliative care: the report of the consensus conference. J Palliat Med. 2009;12:885–904.
16. Puchalski C, Vitillo R, Hull S, Reller N. Improving the spiritual dimension of whole person care: reaching national and international consensus. J Palliat Med. 2014b;17(6):2014.

17. Ray C, Wyatt TR. Religion and spirituality as a cultural asset in medical students. J Relig Health. 2018;57:1062–73.

18. Robinson MR, Thiel MM, Shirkey K, Zurakowski D, Meyer EC. Efficacy of training interprofessional spiritual care generalists. J Palliat Med. 2016;19:814–21.

19. Shand JC. "Existential Fridays"—reflection in action. Pediatr Blood Cancer. 2018;65:e27004.

20. Smith AC, Kleinman S. Managing emotions in medical school: students' contacts with the living and the dead. Soc Psychol Q. 1989;52:56–69.

21. Wasson LT, Cusmano A, Meli L, Louh I, Falzon L, Hampsey M, Young G, Shaffer J, Davidson KW. Association between learning environment interventions and medical student well-being: a systematic review. JAMA. 2016;316:2237–52.

22. Neely D, Minford EJ. Current status of teaching on spirituality in UK medical schools. Med Educ. 2008;42(2):176–82.

23. Balboni TA, Paulk ME, Balboni MJ, Phelps AC, Loggers ET, Wright AA, Block SD, Lewis EF, Peteet JR, Prigerson HG. Provision of spiritual care to patients with advanced cancer: associations with medical care and quality of life near death. J Clin Oncol. 2010;28(3):445–52.

24. Astrow AB, Wexler A, Texeira K, Kai He M, Sulmasy DP. Is failure to meet spiritual needs associated with cancer patients' perceptions of quality of care and their satisfaction with care? J Clin Oncol. 2007;25(36):5753–7.

25. Kaldjian LC, Jekel JF, Friedland G. End-of-life decisions in HIV-positive patients. AIDS. 1998;12(1):103–7.

26. Tsevat J, Sherman SN, McElwee JA, Mandell KL, Simbartl LA, Sonnenberg FA, Fowler FJ Jr. The will to live among HIV-infected patients. Ann Intern Med. 1999;131(3):194.

27. Curlin FA, Lantos JD, Roach CJ, Sellergren SA, Chin MH. Religious characteristics of U.S. physicians. J Gen Intern Med. 2005;20(7):629–34.

28. Puchalski CM, Guenther M. Restoration and re-creation. Curr Opin Support Palliat Care. 2012;6(2):254–8.

29. Puchalski C, Romer AL. Taking a spiritual history allows clinicians to understand patients more fully. J Palliat Med. 2000;3(1):129–37.

Chapter 7
Wellness for All: Diversity, Challenges, and Opportunities to Improve Wellness for Medical Students

Elizabeth Wilson-Anstey, W. Marcus Lambert, and Heather Krog

Introduction

This chapter explores wellness through as many human perspectives as possible. That is to say, this section examines wellness through the lens of diversity. Each medical student has a different perspective on wellness that is informed by that individual's experiences and culture. Nevertheless, those perspectives are plastic and can be shaped by one's environment. Thus, faculty, administrators, students, and all members of the academic medical community have a unique opportunity to build a healthy culture of wellness that is reflective of the diversity of the institution.

E. Wilson-Anstey (✉) · W. M. Lambert
Weill Cornell Medicine, New York, NY, USA
e-mail: eaanstey@med.cornell.edu; wil2009@med.cornell.edu

H. Krog
Cultural Mentor and Inclusion Facilitator, Copenhagen, Denmark

© Springer Nature Switzerland AG 2019
D. Zappetti, J. D. Avery (eds.), *Medical Student Well-Being*,
https://doi.org/10.1007/978-3-030-16558-1_7

To explain why personal, demographic, and cultural characteristics can impact a medical student's view of wellness, we start by presenting a historical perspective of diversity in medicine. The discourse around diversity and inclusion in academic medicine has changed significantly in the past 50 years. In the late 1960s, the tail end of the civil rights movement, a strong focus was placed on multicultural affairs and inequities faced mostly by minorities. At that time, diversity was secondary to the educational mission. Today, however, diversity is a core part of any vibrant medical school's mission and core values. The Association of American Medical Colleges has also noted that diversity embodies inclusiveness, mutual respect, multiple perspectives, and serves as a catalyst for change resulting in health equity. Diverse groups of thinkers approach problems from different points of view, which help to find creative and inclusive solutions to problems. Thus, our responsibility as members of an academic community is to ensure that diversity, inclusion, and equity are a part of the lens through which we evaluate everything around us.

We continue this chapter by presenting challenges to wellness currently faced by medical students from very diverse backgrounds. For example, how does one maintain social wellness while experiencing feelings of isolation? How do you maintain physical wellness when you have very little free time devoted to your own self-care? We touch on challenges faced in seven different dimensions of wellness and how they might differ between students of different races, ethnicities, socioeconomic backgrounds, sexual orientations, and gender identities.

We conclude with concrete steps that medical students can take to lead healthier lives, particularly as they complete their training. Just as we present challenges, we suggest ways to address those challenges found in research literature and through the experiences of the authors and anonymous medical students. Other members of the medical community might find these tips helpful, both in building a supportive community for students and for themselves. This chapter is not intended to be comprehensive by any means. It will simply seek to introduce a new point of view in promoting wellness for all students.

Efforts to Diversify Medical Education

The purpose of this section is to explore the definition of diversity and why it is valued within medical education. With this framework, we can discuss the many different backgrounds of our students and how these backgrounds affect our efforts to achieve wellness for them. Once we understand students' motivations to pursue medicine and why it is important that we train a diverse physician workforce, we may better understand the tools necessary to nurture the success of a diverse student body.

How Is Diversity Defined?

Diversity is defined in several ways. The US Office of Personnel Management, Office of Diversity and Inclusion, defines workforce diversity as:

> A collection of individual attributes that together help agencies pursue organizational objectives efficiently and effectively. These include, but are not limited to, characteristics such as national origin, language, race, color, disability, ethnicity, gender, age, religion, sexual orientation, gender identity, socioeconomic status, veteran status, and family structures. The concept also encompasses differences among people concerning where they are from and where they have lived and their differences of thought and life experiences [1].

The Sullivan Commission on Diversity in the Healthcare Workforce, a group of 16 health, business, higher education, and legal experts and other leaders, defines racial and ethnic diversity in the healthcare workforce as encompassing several characteristics:

1. The representation of all racial and ethnic groups from the community served within a given healthcare agency, institution, or system.
2. The system-wide incorporation of diverse skills, talents, and ideas from those racial and ethnic groups.
3. The sharing of professional development opportunities and resources, as well as responsibilities and power among all racial and ethnic groups and at all levels of a given agency, institution, or system [2].

In this chapter, we define diversity as the representation of individuals coming from backgrounds underrepresented in medicine: Black or African American; Hispanic or Latino; and American Indian or Alaskan Native. We also include other populations traditionally marginalized or underrepresented in the healthcare workforce: first-generation college students; women; those who identify as lesbian, gay, transgender, bisexual, and/or queer; immigrants; individuals with mental or physical disabilities; older individuals; veterans; and those of lower socioeconomic status.

Importance of Diversity in Medical Education

In 2003, the US Supreme Court ruled that there is value to diverse representation in a school or work setting [3]. The Association of American Medical Colleges (AAMC) is a governing body for medical education in the USA and Canada, comprising hundreds of medical schools and teaching hospitals. For over a century, it has been considered a leader within academic medicine, at the forefront of innovation and excellence in training. The organization strives to "cultivate *Human Capital* by enhancing the skills of individuals; build *Organizational Capacity* by improving institutions' ability to use diversity as a driver of excellence; and grow a diverse and culturally-prepared health workforce… [4]." The Group on Student Affairs-Committee on Student Diversity Affairs (COSDA) within the AAMC emphasizes the importance of ensuring diversity within medical education, positing that diversity in medicine enriches the educational environment and reduces healthcare disparities and that a diverse physician workforce is necessary in order to meet the needs of our increasingly diverse population [5]. The Liaison Committee for Medical Education (LCME) of the American Medical Association (AMA) and the AAMC accredits medical education programs in medical schools. This body places a high emphasis on diversity, viewing it to be critically important both to increase the size of the physician workforce and to effectively integrate cultural competence into medical schools' curricula [6].

Individual researchers have also explored the benefits of diversity. Gurin, Dey, Hurtado, and Gurin [7] examined the relationship between the experiences college and university students have with diverse classmates and their educational outcomes. Americano and Bhugra stated that diversity is "valuing the contributions of everyone in society, embracing individual differences and encompassing the full range of social groupings [8]." Results of their analysis indicated that there are educational and civic benefits to Asian American, African American, Hispanic, and White students interacting in the classroom and informal settings. The intermingling of diverse groups of college students promotes positive academic and social outcomes [9, 10]. In addition to racial diversity being educationally significant to students and medical schools, the authors found that a diverse workforce increased the efficiency and effectiveness of organizations.

Beginning in the late 1960s, medical schools established offices of minority affairs solely to address the enrollment and retention of racial and ethnic minority students. During this period, Diversity 1.0 as described by Nivet [11], minority affairs offices were silos running parallel to the other functions of the medical school, research, education, and patient care (Fig. 7.1). Diversity 2.0 was seen as beginning in the 1980s when discussions on the importance of having a diverse, culturally competent, and culturally sensitive physician workforce and linking it to the improvement of patient health care and the reduction of healthcare disparities began [11–17]. Medical schools then developed curricula to improve the skills and attributes of students as they interacted with a diverse patient population [18]. Medical student diversity, physician workforce diversity, and diversity in the curriculum form are seen as important components for excellence in medical education. Offices of minority affairs which focused solely on the needs of students from racially and ethnically diverse backgrounds have now become offices of diversity and inclusion supporting the wellness of a wider and more diverse medical student population.

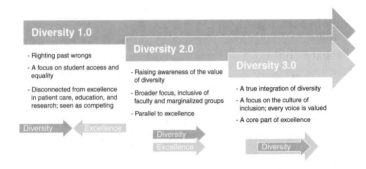

FIGURE 7.1 The transformation of diversity in medical education

Diversity in the US Population and Medical Schools

In 2018, the total US population was 328 million [19]. By 2060, that number is projected to increase to 404 million. As presented in Table 7.1, of the 404 million, 60.7 million (15.0%) are projected to be Black or African American; 5.6 million (1.4%) American Indian and Alaska Native; 36.8 million (9.1%) Asian; and 111.2 million (27.5%) Hispanic or Latino, the largest percentage increase among all groups [20] (Table 7.1).

In December 2018, the AAMC reported an increase in applicants and matriculants to medical school that identified as Black or African American (by 4.0% to 5164 and 4.6% to 1856, respectively), and American Indian or Alaska Native (by 10.0% to 559, and 6.3% to 218, respectively) [21]. In 2018, 351 military service members applying for medical school admission stated they were veterans, and 175 were on active duty [22]. Individuals with disabilities are also adding to the diversity of the medical student body [23, 24].

As stated earlier, diversity is increasingly being recognized as an important and core component for excellence in training medical students, and in building a diverse physician workforce that provides care to a diverse population. Therefore, in preparing for a US population that is growing

TABLE 7.1 Projected population by race and Hispanic origin for the USA: 2016 to 2060

Race and ethnicity	2016 Numbers in thousands	2016 Percent	2060 Numbers in thousands	2060 Percent	Change, 2016–2060
Total	323,128		404,483		
One race	314,648	97.4%	379,228	93.8%	−3.6%
White	248,503	76.9%	275,014	68.0%	−8.9%
Non-Hispanic White	197,970	61.3%	179,162	44.3%	−17%
Black or African American	43,001	13.3%	60,690	15.0%	+1.7%
American Indian and Alaska Native	4055	1.3%	5583	1.4%	+0.1%
Asian	18,319	5.7%	36,815	9.1%	+3.4%
Native Hawaiian and other Pacific Islander	771	0.2%	1125	0.3%	+0.1%
Two or more races	8480	2.6%	25,255	6.2%	+3.6%
Hispanic or Latino origin[a]	57,470	17.8%	111,216	27.5%	+9.7%

[a]Not a race

racially and ethnically and includes a greater number of veterans, individuals with disabilities, and first-generation medical students entering medical schools, student affairs professionals need to create an inclusive on-campus environment where all students can thrive.

Moving forward, there will be important questions institutions must ask in order to properly embrace, nurture, and benefit from the rising diversity within medical education. For example, medical schools have moved beyond the narrowly focused definition of diversity, one's race and ethnicity, to include a student's socioeconomic status, sexual orientation, gender identity, disability, gender, and veteran status. Do students from such diverse backgrounds face unique challenges that affect their wellness? How do different life experiences affect the wellness of students in medical school? What types of activities, opportunities, or programs should medical schools have in order for students not to feel excluded, but included and valued at the institution? How could student affairs professionals support and assist medical students from diverse backgrounds adjust to a new, high-pressured environment where they are expected to achieve academically? Creating and building a supportive community of respect, and understanding is a start.

Challenges Faced by Students from Historically Underrepresented and Marginalized Populations

The healthcare challenges we face as a society, including an aging population and a rapidly shifting system of delivery, demand all of the resources that we can marshal. We need people from all over the world, with different perspectives, different abilities, and different approaches, to help us discover new solutions. (Augustine M.K. Choi, M.D., Stephen and Suzanne Weiss Dean, Weill Cornell Medicine)

Just as perceptions of diversity and excellence must transform from a parallel mission (Diversity 2.0) to diversity as a core part of excellence (Diversity 3.0) [11], diversity must be seen in the same way as an integral part of promoting and sustaining wellness. For most medical schools and academic medical centers, promoting wellness requires a cultural change that cannot be devoid of diversity. This means that wellness should be both inclusive and adapted when necessary. For example, some human resource departments will incentivize their employees to take the stairs instead of an elevator with gift cards, prizes, or event tickets. While this is a great way to promote overall physical activity and wellness, a *Step Challenge* may not be accessible to all who would be interested in participating. By incorporating people of all abilities (perhaps through a *Movement Challenge*), a cultural shift is made that maximizes the benefit of the wellness effort for everyone involved (Fig. 7.2).

Wellness that incorporates diversity through the lens of specialized support is also essential. For example, lactation

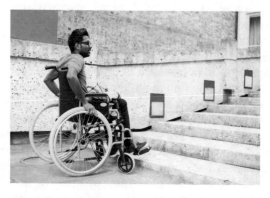

FIGURE 7.2 Common barriers to participation experienced by people with physical disabilities

rooms can provide nursing mothers support as they transition back to the workplace. Promoting wellness often means finding ways to address challenges unique to or more prevalent in certain groups and populations. In this section, we will cover many of the most common challenges faced by medical students from underrepresented and marginalized groups. Underrepresentation in medicine refers to racial and ethnic populations that are disproportionately represented in medicine. We will dive deep into the experiences unique to these populations. We will also explore challenges faced by other traditionally marginalized populations (e.g., women; first-generation students; people who identify as lesbian, gay, transgender, bisexual, and/or queer; immigrants; individuals with mental or physical disabilities; older individuals; veterans; and those of lower socioeconomic status). Many of the challenges that face members of one or more of these groups can—singularly or in combination—be the very thing that threatens their sense of wellness and derails their academic excellence. We will explore the challenges that students from traditionally underrepresented and marginalized groups can face across seven dimensions: physical, emotional, financial, social, spiritual, intellectual, and occupational.

Physical wellness includes a number of healthy behaviors including adequate exercise, proper nutrition, and abstaining from harmful habits such as drug use and alcohol abuse. Some students may find maintaining healthy diets and regular exercise challenging for several reasons. First, the demands of the medical school curriculum leave little time for leisure activities. For many students who hold significant obligations to family, such as taking care of a sick parent, sending money back home, or even raising a family of their own, their "free time" can often compete with self-care. Exercising, eating healthy and periodic meals, and getting the proper amount of sleep all have to be intentionally scheduled into a routine, and sacrificing the time to do so can be a challenge for some students, particularly from diverse backgrounds.

> Wellness committees often instruct students to continue with a hobby or to seek out new pleasurable activities. But with no financial support and an unusual family dynamic, my limited free time was spent working or supporting my family. There was no time to employ self-care techniques. (Medical Student)

As stated earlier, we anonymously collected student anecdotes about wellness from around the country. One student noted, "often times we are faced with the responsibility of caring for our families. As a child of immigrants, my parents rely on me to help them navigate the healthcare system, education system, etc. Though, I've left home, I am still in charge of ensuring my younger brother is studying for the SATs, checking his grades online, and corresponding with his school counselor." Another medical student noted, "wellness committees often instruct students to continue with a hobby or to seek out new pleasurable activities. But with no financial support and an unusual family dynamic, my limited free time was spent working or supporting my family. There was no time to employ self-care techniques."

Second, not all students have the financial means to afford access to the type of physical wellness that they might prefer such as gym memberships. While most medical students have access to workout facilities on campus, many may find local gym memberships to be a financial sacrifice that is not worth the price despite their offering a more diverse array of exercise activities. The same can be said for the purchase of healthy food options of their preference. It is no secret that food prices pose a significant barrier for anyone who is trying to balance good nutrition with affordability. When incomes drop and budgets shrink, it has been shown that food choices shift toward cheaper, more energy-dense foods [25]. Despite financial aid, many medical students have a small amount money with which to balance normal living expenses with extra expenses like traveling home for the holidays, paying for test preparation materials, or supporting family in need. Students from low socioeconomic and other diverse backgrounds can find themselves sacrificing a lot, whether it be time or money, to maintain physical wellness.

Another challenge to consider in the dimension of physical wellness is the diversity of the activities. For many students, activities often associated with reducing stress such as yoga, meditation, mindfulness techniques, etc. are new cultural phenomena for many students of underrepresented backgrounds. One student notes, "wellness techniques employed by my institution are new to me and thus wellness sessions are always a learning experience more so than stress reducers." When medical institutions or current students promote wellness activities, they can often lack the cultural diversity representative of their place of residence or even their class.

> Family Day was an annual event held by the medical school to provide parents and friends with a glimpse of medical student life. However, for student's like me it was just another source of stress. Many of my classmates had at least one physician parent for whom Family Day could be an opportunity to discuss the new challenges medical students faced. Almost all the students had college educated parents who had familiarity with graduate level programs. But if no one in your immediate family had anything beyond a GED, your concern became 'would my family feel comfortable participating in the mock PBL sessions'? What about if your family doesn't speak English? (Medical Student)

Emotional wellness is arguably the most impacted dimension of wellness for underrepresented and marginalized populations. Students from diverse backgrounds not only face a number of external challenges and stresses from being members of a particular group or identity but can internalize emotions or feelings around adverse experiences related to identity. For example, minority students are more likely to report that their race/ethnicity has adversely affected their medical school experience [26]. Countless times Hispanic or Black/African American medical students, residents, and physicians are mistaken for the janitor or other hospital support staff, despite wearing identification, a white coat and/or a stethoscope.

Medical students from other marginalized groups have reported that they have experienced similar microaggressions, which are short repeated behaviors or experiences that express a prejudice attitude toward a member of a marginalized group. Most microaggressions are thought to be subtle, indirect, or unintentional, as opposed to microassaults which are conscious and discriminatory actions. Microassaults can happen to medical students, too, particularly when dealing with patients. In any of the above cases, underrepresented minority medical students have to learn to navigate others' unconscious biases more often than not. Yet, members of these groups often lack the tools to react to situations that challenge parts of their identity. Many even fear succumbing to stereotypes about their social group, known as stereotype threat, causing them to change their actions, behaviors, and/or suppressing negative thoughts and emotions [27].

Microaggressions are also common among students who identify as LGBTQ+ (lesbian, gay, bisexual, transgender, or queer). Sexual orientation microaggressions are thought to threaten LGBTQ students' academic development and emotional well-being [28]. Women, too, can face enormous bias in the form of microaggressions or simply discriminatory acts. In every marginalized group, these experiences have an opportunity to impact the emotional wellness of the student.

In addition to microaggressions, some medical students face imposter phenomena or imposter syndrome. They question their accomplishments and success even in the face of information that indicates the opposite is true. This can lead to feelings that they are acting as an *imposter*, and that they are not inherently as qualified as their classmates. This most often occurs at transitionary periods and is heightened at moments where students face new challenges, including the start of medical school or residency. One student characterized it like this, "I don't think it's the fault of anyone in particular but as someone from a diverse background, there was a huge chip on my shoulder. Am I actually smart, capable and deserve to be here or am I fulfilling a quota? Do my professors believe I'm great or just great for someone of my ethnicity? No one can provide you with self-esteem, but I don't think wellness efforts addressed the difficulties posed when you are the only member of your race in every setting."

> Am I actually smart, capable and deserve to be here or am I fulfilling a quota? (Medical Student)

The next dimension of wellness is one that is often treated as a necessary precondition for other forms of wellness. While financial stress certainly impacts many of the other dimensions, *financial wellness* implies not just having money but knowing how to manage it. By definition, students from low socioeconomic backgrounds face income and occupation challenges that impact their education and access to resources. These students are often very tied to family, having to care for siblings and parents, both financially and educationally. A student notes, "during the holidays, I witness my peers fill with excitement to go home and visit family. I simply do not share the same excitement, because I know that when I'm home I will inevitably pick up the responsibilities I had before I left home to attend medical school."

In many cases, these students cannot afford to make financial mistakes. When they experience financial difficulties, they don't have parents or family members to turn to for help. When they only have five dollars left for the week, diet becomes dollar pizza or Ramen noodles, and physical, emotional, and social wellness become secondary. One student shares, "…a significant part of wellness could be derived from social gatherings. Going to the local pub or the Halloween party was an easy, cheap way to socialize. For more costly events like the school ski trip, I had to choose between spending time with my class or paying for a UWorld question bank that was practically required for the clerkship years. It's really difficult to get the social support from your peers when you literally cannot afford to spend time with them."

Social wellness is an integral part of overall wellness for medical students, but for underrepresented students, international students, and others, medical school could mean fitting into an entirely new social community, different from ones that may have been left behind. Dr. Richard Friedman, a professor of Clinical Psychiatry at Weill Cornell Medicine, often asks students, "How many of you went to college in New York City?" and very few hands go up. He then says, "Most of you left your close friends and social network behind, so it's natural to feel stressed and lonely." Dr. Gus Kappler, author of *Welcome Home From Vietnam, Finally: A Vietnam Trauma Surgeon's Memoir*, emphasizes the importance of student affairs professionals recognizing military veterans who often have vastly different backgrounds from their civilian classmates. "The military is created to run as cohesive units," he notes. Once outside of that community, Kappler states that many military veterans "struggle to reintegrate back into the society. They feel like outsiders" [29].

Isolation and difficulty connecting with peers is a challenge faced by minority and non-minority students alike. However, minority students have also reported feeling isolated from faculty and their family. Furthermore, underrepresented minorities also find themselves in situations where they are the only minority or one of very few minorities in academic medical centers. This lack of critical mass affects exposure to role models, mentorship, and even the level of support that they receive from their peers. Many medical schools do not have enough Black or Hispanic students to successfully run a Black student club (i.e., SNMA) or Hispanic student club (i.e., LMSA). They often find themselves banning together to form an umbrella minority or diversity group just to find community among themselves.

Immigrants and children of immigrants to the USA may have similar challenges, vastly different cultural expectations, or face a level of stress over immigration policy that probably deserves its own wellness dimension. Some undocumented students, for example, live their lives with the possibility that at any moment, they or a member of their family could be deported back to a country where they may have little familiarity or sense of safety. Thus, it remains important to examine the experiences people have in their social communities and how that affects their wellness.

Spiritual wellness is also tied to social wellness. For many students starting medical school, they leave behind religious communities, practices, and traditions. Many have to find new places to pray, people in which to celebrate holidays, ways to continue their diet, and new communities to join. For many students, spiritual wellness is an integral part of their overall well-being. If access and resources to maintain this well-being are limited, it may present challenges to those students' academic progress as well. Orthodox Jewish students, for example, might find it difficult in some parts of the USA to find kosher foods or a religious community nearby. Students of some faiths may receive microaggressions and comments that make them feel unwelcome. These challenges and overall lack of access to religious norms can affect the wellness of many medical students.

Students who do not prescribe to a traditional religion also find a need for spiritual wellness. Spiritual wellness is simply defined by a set of guiding beliefs, principles, or values that help to direct a student's life. These beliefs help to provide a sense of meaning and purpose for students. They are an outlet during times of stress, and a source of constancy when life is dynamic and changing. It is important that students recognize and determine the value of spiritual wellness in their lives and how it fits in their normal routines.

Intellectual wellness can also be a source of well-being for students. With creative, stimulating mental activities, students can find ways to relieve stress and maintain homeostasis. Students from diverse backgrounds, however, may find their intellectual interests informed heavily by their culture and may not be fully represented or even embraced by others in their academic community. A book club that never diverges from Eastern European literature may not be welcoming to students from diverse backgrounds. Lack of diversity within the medical school curriculum can also be challenging to students, especially when only one or two students speak about the concern.

Finally, *occupational wellness* invokes a right to explore careers and work that makes students happy. A diverse physician population is an important aspect in addressing health-care disparities among patients. Increasing the number of underrepresented minority physicians in the USA has been posited as a strategy for improving the health of minority and underserved communities. However, students should not feel pressured to enter primary care because of their background or treated differently because they are the only woman in their specialty. Similarly, for service to the institution and community, one's background should not define the level of their service. Students sometimes feel what is known as the *Black and Brown tax* or *Diversity tax*, when they are con-stantly asked to do service-related activities because of their background. This could lead to burnout, which continues to be a serious threat to physician well-being.

Call to Action: Improve the Wellness of Your Diverse Medical Student Community

So far in this chapter, we have presented challenges across seven dimensions (physical, emotional, financial, social, spiri-tual, intellectual, and occupational) faced by students from underrepresented and marginalized groups. In this section, we will reconsider these challenges as opportunities for improvement. While this guide is written for the medical stu-dent, improving medical student wellness is a charge for the entire medical community. We are better equipped to improve each other's overall sense of wellness as a community rather than as individuals. While reading through the following sug-gestions, students and student affairs professionals should consider how to apply these tips to their own community.

Physical wellness—Promoting regular exercise and proper nutrition should be an initiative of the entire academic com-munity. Medical students should encourage healthy physical behavior among their peers. Find accountability partners to hold each other to your goals. Taking one-minute wellness breaks are quick, simple ways to improve health and wellness at no financial cost. For example, stay hydrated by drinking water; take deep breaths; go outside into the sunshine; give yourself a mini-massage by rubbing your hands, feet, and shoulders; and do jumping jacks or push-ups if you are able [30]. Taking ten-minute wellness breaks to practice yoga or stretching activities, call a supportive relative or partner, listen to calming music, or meditation are other ways to improve wellness [31]. Students should feel comfortable finding ways to reduce stress through dance, playing music, and other healthy activities that are reflective of their cultures.

Administrators should ensure that medical students have free access to well-maintained gym facilities on campus that are easily accessible by individuals with a physical disability. A variety of healthy foods and sensitivities to allergies should be taken into consideration when meals are catered. Imagine how much we can promote healthy habits by simply ordering more healthy foods at the next workshop or seminar? Remember, however, to include foods from various cultures. This helps to build an inclusive community and assists students in having a sense of belonging at the institution.

Emotional wellness—Both students and administrators must remain aware of the emotional challenges that are both obvious and hidden in academic community. This vigilance for emotional imbalance can be difficult to maintain, especially for students under stress. As one student puts it, "with the competitive culture of medical school, admitting you're having problems of any sort . . . is tension laden" [32]. Yet, awareness from the entire community is the first step. Students check-in on your peers. Administrators check-in on students. Student affairs professionals in particular must be sensitive to challenges that diverse students encounter.

When a challenge is identified, know your resources. The office of medical student diversity and inclusion, or its equivalent, is a place on campus where students should feel they can go to express their concerns, feel welcome, and get their concerns addressed. Students from diverse backgrounds should not be shy about seeking out medical school-provided mental health services. These services are confidential and can often make a tremendous difference in academic productivity. Overcoming any stigma associated with mental health services can be one of the largest challenges faced in under-represented populations. It is, therefore, important for faculty and staff to be culturally sensitive, knowledgeable of the backgrounds from which diverse students are coming and be willing to work with all students so they can thrive. The medical school should actively take affirmative steps to remove barriers that hinder the emotional well-being of its students.

The emotional wellness toolkit assembled by the National Institutes of Health provides six strategies to improve one's emotional health: (1) Brighten one's outlook by being resilient and having fewer negative emotions; (2) learn healthy ways to reduce stress; (3) get quality sleep; (4) cope with loss; (5) strengthen social connections; (6) and practice mindfulness [33]. While these strategies are *easier said than done*, recognizing these strategies and incorporating them into one's goals is the first step. Second, students should seek out community. Join an interest group of like-minded individuals and become involved with outreach activities to communities similar to your own. Giving back to others can keep you focused on your career path, and help you remember why you chose to become physicians. Finally, take advantage of safe spaces to discuss microaggressions and micro-assaults that you experience can help to confirm or clarify your perception of what caused the harm. Discuss strategies to handle such assaults if they reoccur.

Financial wellness—A student having to support family members financially or emotionally while in medical school is taxing. Medical schools could address this financial burden by creating an environment where students facing such challenges would feel comfortable revealing such hardships. As stated earlier, medical students may be reluctant to divulge such situations in an environment where many of their peers come from wealthier backgrounds. Students from lower socioeconomic backgrounds may feel embarrassed and out of place. Medical schools should create a community where such challenges faced by students are discussed and take steps to address those difficulties. Schools should also actively recruit a diverse student body so that first-year students could find others in their class from similar backgrounds. This could reduce isolation and loneliness. Creating safe spaces where students can tell their stories and converse openly and respectfully has the potential to increase understanding, to reveal commonalities among peers, and to foster a sense of belonging.

Adequate financial aid should be made available for students. The director of financial aid should become aware of and understand the financial challenges faced by the first generation or students from financially disadvantaged backgrounds at their institutions. Debt management workshops should be held in a culturally sensitive way, so that students gain the most from the interactions and are not offended or feel embarrassed by their lack of knowledge of how to manage their finances, or lack of funds to take part in activities that are not free of charge. Institutions should consider subsidizing the cost of cultural events. The financial assistance would enable students with limited funds to engage more easily with community activities.

Regardless of the degree to which students are concerned with their finances, it is important for them to have an overview of their personal financial situation. Students should be aware of the AAMC's resources for financial wellness. Among other tools, this program includes financial calculators, articles, and videos to create a budget, track spending, create financial goals, and enhance their financial knowledge about credit, financial planning, money management, as well as the opportunity to enroll in the association's financial wellness program [34].

Social wellness—All students should be encouraged to take deliberate steps to care for themselves, thereby improving social wellness. Through self-reflection, and recognition of their social needs, students with different experiences could thrive in a medical school community that embraces diversity. Students from diverse backgrounds feel included and have a sense of belonging when their cultures are recognized and validated by others. There are advantages to learning together and listening to each other. Students should consider seeking classmates with similar experiences and form study groups with those whom they are comfortable. Doing so promotes "a culture of acceptance and eagerness to learn from one another will foster a collaborative and supportive environment. This could serve to decrease the sense of isolation felt by minority medical students as reported in some studies" [35]. Joining a national organization that has local chapters can help a student to develop a sense of belonging and strengthen the sense of community on campus. Some examples include the Student National Medical Association, Latino Medical Students Association, Association of Native American Medical Students, and the Students Veterans Association. If a group of interest does not exist on campus, students should seek advice from their office of Student Affairs or Community Service Office on how one can be established.

As noted earlier in the chapter, 351 military service members applying for medical school admission stated they were veterans, and 175 were on active duty [22]. Having student activities during *Joining Forces Wellness Week* [36] in recognition of Veterans Day, for example, would be one way to acknowledge a marginalized individual within the medical school. Doing so as a community can increase cultural competency and can educate other students about healthcare needs unique to veterans, military service members, and their families. An inspiring example of this is when the AAMC celebrated the *Fifth Annual Joining Forces Wellness Week* highlighting healthcare needs of veterans, military service members, and their families in 2016.

Beyond events highlighting individuals of specific backgrounds, creating safe spaces where students can tell their stories and converse openly and respectfully has the potential to increase understanding. When interacting with military veterans, Kappler [29] stresses the importance of getting to know the person by saying, "Welcome home" and not "thanks for your service." That statement is considered trite. "How can I help you, tell me your story" lets military service members feel that they matter, and someone is willing to listen to an account of their experiences Kappler [29]. (For additional resources, consider contacting your local chapter of Students Veterans of America [37].) This example of inclusivity should be considered for students of many backgrounds in order to bolster social wellness.

Spiritual wellness—Both for their own sake and for the sake of their patients, students should be encouraged to develop and maintain their spiritual wellness. Whether or not students consider themselves to be spiritual persons, tending to their spiritual well-being helps prepare them to treat spiritually minded patients. "Studies indicate patients want their physicians to have knowledge of their spiritual beliefs to facilitate better understanding of them as individuals, as well as help physicians understand patients' decision-making" [38].

The spiritual practices of a diverse student body should be respected and uplifted by the medical school community. The medical school core curriculum must provide all students with the knowledge and skills that would help to develop their attitudes to care for a diverse patient population. Many premedical students from backgrounds underrepresented in medicine choose to become physicians in order to improve health care for underserved populations and to reduce healthcare disparities. "From health promotion interventions to day-to-day interactions with health care providers, spirituality can be a useful means of connecting with patients for whom this is an important aspect of life" [39].

Intellectual wellness—Students should be encouraged to seek faculty mentors. "Mentors can model professionalism and ethical behavior to mentees, while mentees can inspire mentors to remain true to their ideals and remind them of their original calling to practice medicine. When mentors and mentees are from dissimilar generations or backgrounds, both parties can benefit from an expanding awareness of differences" [40, 41]. This is a prime example of diversity being the core of excellence as, here, it enhances the mutual benefit of engaging in and nurturing a mentor-mentee relationship. Students should also seek upperclassmen for advice. They can provide valuable insight into what is to come during the medical training journey. They can also serve as mentors in the same way that mentees can serve as mentors for students in the future.

Recalling the challenge presented by the lack of diversity within of the medical school curriculum, there is a real opportunity to create more space for intellectual inquiry and curiosity. An infusion of more diverse perspectives into the core curriculum can expand areas of study that can pique the interest of faculty and student alike. Realizing this opportunity rests upon the faculty, staff, and administration who have the responsibility of organizing and delivering medical training, as well as the authority and decision-making power to affect change. Medical schools should assess their curriculum to ensure that knowledge, skills, and attitudes pertaining to diversity and cultural competency are addressed throughout the curriculum.

Occupational wellness—Burnout, or the "loss of enthusiasm for work, feelings of cynicism, and a low sense of personal accomplishment [42]" continues to be a serious threat to physician well-being and, therefore, to patient care. Black and Asian female physicians have reported experiencing bias from patients and the public at large who question their ability and qualifications to be physicians [43, 44]. The number of physicians suffering from burnout is increasing: 40% in 2013, and 51% in 2017 [45]. Given this reality, during training, all students must consider taking stock of their tendency toward burning out. In this regard, measuring one's occupational wellness according to the Maslach Burnout Inventory [46] is instructive, as it measures both the nature (emotional exhaustion, depersonalization, and personal accomplishment) and degree (low, moderate, and high) of burnout.

Now, while there is limited data available regarding how to best address trainee burnout, it has been identified that the learning and work environment, rather than individual attributes, are the major drivers of burnout [47]. It is, therefore, important for medical school faculty, staff, and administration to help create a more nurturing learning environment for students in training.

Finally, in order to improve occupational wellness and to avoid burnout, Black or African American, Hispanic or

Latino, and Native American medical students should be mindful of the diversity tax and the balance between service and studies. A good place to start this discussion would be in their Offices of Diversity. This office liaises between medical students and the school's faculty and leadership. Therefore, the staff can listen with an understanding ear and direct you to relevant students, faculty, staff, support spaces, etc.

Summary

Diversity and inclusion are receiving increased attention within the medical community and looking at wellness from this wider lens revealed different challenges faced by individuals depending on their background. Thus, we see that diversity and inclusion are a core aspect of wellness (Fig. 7.3).

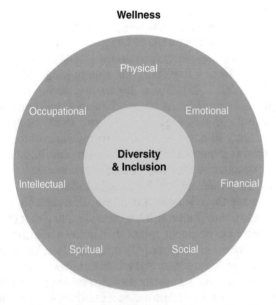

FIGURE 7.3 Diversity and inclusion are at the core of wellness

In this chapter's call to action, we concluded with ideas for actions that can be taken to improve wellness in medical student training. Suggestions were made within each of the seven dimensions of wellness, and, where relevant, they were directed toward medical school faculty, staff, and administration. These recommendations are, admittedly, neither exhaustive nor comprehensive. However, this is stated resting upon the understanding that improving medical students' wellness is a community-wide issue that requires time and sustained commitment.

References

1. U.S. Office of Personnel Management Office of Diversity and Inclusion. Government-wide diversity and inclusion strategic plan 2011 (2011). Retrieved from http://www.opm.gov/policy-data-oversight/diversity-and-inclusion/reports/government-widedistrategicplan.pdf
2. Sullivan Commission. Missing persons: minorities in the health professions, a report of the Sullivan Commission on diversity in the healthcare workforce. Washington, DC: Sullivan Commission; 2004. Retrieved from http://www.aacn.nche.edu/Media/pdf/SullivanReport.pdf
3. Grutter v. Bollinger, 539 U.S. 306 (2003). Retrieved from http://supreme.justia.com/cases/federal/us/539/306/case.html
4. Association of American Medical Colleges (AAMC). About the AAMC. Washington, DC: Association of American Medical Colleges (AAMC); 2018. Retrieved from https://www.aamc.org/about
5. Association of American Medical Colleges (AAMC). Charge of the GSA-Committee on Student Diversity Affairs (COSDA). Washington, DC: Association of American Medical Colleges (AAMC); 2018. Retrieved from https://www.aamc.org/download/484190/data/cosda-charge.pdf
6. Liaison Committee on Medical Education (LCME). Functions and structure of a medical school: standards for accreditation of medical education programs leading to the M.D. degree. Diversity pipeline programs and partnerships (2018, March). Retrieved from http://lcme.org/publications/

7. Gurin P, Dey DL, Hurtado S, Gurin G. Diversity and higher education: theory and impact on educational outcomes. Harv Educ Rev. 2002;72(3):330–5. Retrieved from https://igr.umich.edu/files/igr/Diversity%20and%20Higher%20Education.pdf

8. Americano A, Bhugra D. Dealing with diversity. In: Swanwick T, editor. Understanding medical education: evidence, theory and practice; 2013. p. 445–54. https://doi.org/10.1002/9781118472361.ch31.

9. Astin AW. What matters is college. San Francisco: Jossey-Bass; 1993.

10. Antonio AL, Chang MJ, Hakuta K, Kenny DA, Levin S, Milem JF. Effects of racial diversity on complete thinking in college students. Psychol Sci. 2004;15(8):507–10.

11. Nivet M. Diversity 3.0: a necessary systems upgrade. Acad Med. 2011:1487–9. https://doi.org/10.1097/ACM.0b013e3182351f79.

12. Betancourt JR. Cultural competence and medical education: many names many perspectives one goal. Acad Med. 2006:499–501. https://doi.org/10.1097/01.ACM.0000225211.77088.cb.

13. Betancourt JR, Green AR, Carrillo JE, Ananeh-Firempong O. Defining cultural competence: a practical framework for addressing racial/ethnic disparities in health and healthcare. Public Health Rep. 2003;118(4):293–302. Retrieved from http://www.ncbi.nlm.nih.gov/pmc/articles/PMC1497553/

14. Betancourt JR, Green AR, Carrillo JE, Park ER. Cultural competence and healthcare disparities: key perspectives and trends. Health Aff. 2005:499–505. https://doi.org/10.1377/hlthaff.24.2.499.

15. Cohen JJ, Gabriel BA, Terrell C. The case for diversity in the healthcare workforce. Health Aff. 2002:90–102. https://doi.org/10.1377/hlthaff.21.5.90.

16. Institute of Medicine (IOM). In: Smedley BD, Stith AY, Nelson AR, editors. Unequal treatment: confronting racial and ethnic disparities in healthcare. Washington, DC: National Academies Press; 2003.

17. Steinbrook R. Diversity in medicine. N Engl J Med. 1996:1327–8. https://doi.org/10.1056/NEJM199605163342011.

18. Lie DA, Boker J, Crandall S, DeGannes CN, Elliott D, Henderson P, Kodjo C, Seng L. Revising the Tool for Assessing Cultural Competence Training (TACCT) for curriculum evaluation: findings derived from seven US schools and expert consensus (2008, Jan 1). Retrieved from https://www.ncbi.nlm.nih.gov/pubmed/19756238

19. U.S. Census Bureau. Population clock December 13, 2018. U.S. Census Bureau; 2019. Retrieved from https://www.census.gov

20. U.S. Census Bureau. 2017 National Population Projections Tables (2018, September 6). Retrieved from https://www.census.gov/data/tables/2017/demo/popproj/2017-summary-tables.html

21. Association of American Medical Colleges (AAMC). Women were majority or U.S. medical school applicants in 2018. AAMC News. Washington, DC: Association of American Medical Colleges (AAMC); 2018. Retrieved from https://news.aamc.org/press-releases/article/applicant-data-2018/

22. Association of American Medical Colleges (AAMC). Applying as a veteran or current military member. Washington, DC: Association of American Medical Colleges (AAMC); 2018. Retrieved from https://students-residents.aamc.org/applying-medical-school/article/applying-veteran-or-current-military-member/

23. Association of American Medical Colleges (AAMC). Women were majority or U.S. medical school applicants in 2018. AAMC News. Washington, DC: Association of American Medical Colleges (AAMC); 2018. Retrieved from https://news.aamc.org/diversity/article/paving-way-med-students-physicians-disabilities/

24. Watson JR, Hutchens SH. Medical students with disabilities: a generation of practice. Washington, DC: Association of American Medical Colleges; 2005. Retrieved from https://members.aamc.org/eweb/upload/Medical%20Students%20with%20Disabilities%20A%20Generation%202005.pdf

25. Drewnowski A, Eichelsdoerfer P. Can low-income Americans afford a healthy diet? Nutr Today. 2010;44(6):246–9. https://doi.org/10.1097/NT.0b013e3181c29f79.

26. Dyrbye LN, Thomas MR, Eacker A, Harper W, Massie FS Jr, Power DV, et al. Race, ethnicity, and medical student well-being in the United States. Arch Intern Med. 2007;167(19):2103–9. https://doi.org/10.1001/archinte.167.19.2103.

27. Aronson J, Burgess D, Phelan SM, Juarez L. Unhealthy interactions: the role of stereotype threat in health disparities. Am J Public Health. 2013;103(1):50–6. https://doi.org/10.2105/AJPH.2012.300828.

28. Nadal KL, Issa M, Leon J, Meterko V, Wideman M, Wong Y. Sexual orientation microaggressions: "death by a thousand cuts" for lesbian, gay, and bisexual youth. J LGBT Youth. 2011;8(3):234–59. https://doi.org/10.1080/19361653.2011.584204.

29. Kappler G (2018, December 18). Personal interview.

30. Walters J. 60-Second health and fitness boosters (2010). Retrieved from https://www.sparkpeople.com/resource/wellness_articles. asp?id=1557
31. Editors of Prevention. 100 Ways to change your life in 10 minutes or less (2014). Retrieved from https://www.prevention.com/life/a20440708/10-minute-health-and-wellness-tips/
32. Association of American Medical Colleges (AAMC). Paving the way for medical students, physicians with disabilities. Washington, DC: Association of American Medical Colleges (AAMC); 2018. Retrieved from https://news.aamc.org/diversity/article/paving-way-med-students-physicians-disabilities/
33. National Institutes of Health. Emotional wellness toolkit. Bethesda: National Institutes of Health; 2018. Retrieved from https://www.nih.gov/health-information/emotional-wellness-toolkit
34. Association of American Medical Colleges. Financial wellness for medical school and beyond. Washington, DC: Association of American Medical Colleges; 2018. Retrieved from https://aamc-financialwellness.com/index.cfm
35. Editorial Board. Minority attrition and burnout among US medical students, J Stud Natl Med Assoc. (2011). Retrieved from http://jsnma.org/article/minority-attrition-and-burnout-among-us-medical-students/
36. Association of American Medical Colleges (AAMC). Fifth Annual Joining Forces Wellness Week Highlights Health Care Needs of Veterans, Military Service Members, and Their Families (2016). Retrieved from https://news.aamc.org/press-releases/article/joining-forces-wellness-week-2016/
37. Students Veterans of American (2018). Retrieved from https://studentveterans.org
38. Isaac KS, Hay JL, Lubetkin EI. Incorporating spirituality in primary care. J Relig Health. 2016;55(3):1065–77. https://doi.org/10.1007/s10943-016-0190-2.
39. McCord G, Gilchrist VJ, Grossman SD, King BD, McCormick KF, Oprandi AM, et al. Discussing spirituality with patients: a rational and ethical approach. Ann Fam Med. 2004;2(4):356–61. https://doi.org/10.1370/afm.71.
40. Choi AMK, Moon JE, Steinecke A, Prescott JE. Developing a culture of mentorship to strengthen academic medical Centers. Acad Med. 2018; https://doi.org/10.1097/ACM.0000000000002498.
41. Waljee JF, Chopra V, Saint S. Mentoring millennials. J Am Med Assoc. 2018;319(15):1547–8. https://doi.org/10.1001/jama.2018.3804.

42. Shanafelt TD, Boone S, Tan L, Dyrbye LN, Sotile W, Satele D, et al. Burnout and satisfaction with work-life balance among US physicians relative to the general US population. Arch Intern Med. 2012;172(18):1377–85. https://doi.org/10.1001/archinternmed.2012.3199.

43. Swartz A. Survey finds black, Asian and women doctors are more likely to face bias – from their own patients. *Mic.* (2017, October 19). Retrieved from https://mic.com/articles/185399/survey-finds-black-asian-and-women-doctors-are-more-likely-to-face-bias-from-their-own-patients#.GXC6ZLxaH

44. Emery, C. (Producer), Emery, C. (Director). (2016). Black women in medicine [Documentary] U.S.: URU The Right To Be, Inc.

45. Peckham C. Bias, burnout, race: what physicians told us about the issues. *Medscape.* (2017). Retrieved from https://www.medscape.com/viewarticle/873985

46. McClafferty H. Abbreviated Maslach Burnout inventory. Physician health and well being: The art and science of self-care in medicine (2014). Retrieved from https://www.nzgp-webdirectory.co.nz/site/nzgp-webdirectory2/files/pdfs/forms/soim_abbreviated_maslach_burnout_inventory.pdf

47. Dyrbye L, Shanafelt T. A narrative review on burnout experienced by medical students and residents. Med Educ. 2016;50(2016):132–49. https://doi.org/10.1111/medu.12927.

Chapter 8
Financial Wellness for Medical Students

James M. Dahle

Financial Wellness for Medical Students

Financial literacy and planning are critical components of wellness for all physicians, including those in training. Being a physician is stressful enough without adding the stresses that come from inadequate financial knowledge, planning, and resources. Medical students are in a terrible financial situation. Not only do they have very limited income, if any at all, but thanks to the rapidly rising cost of tuition, a traditional medical student is likely to have annual liabilities exceeding the sum total of all of the money they have earned in their entire life!

Medical school tuition, like that of most undergraduate and graduate educational institutions, has been rising at double the rate of inflation for the last two or three decades. According to the AAMC, the median cost of tuition, fees, and health insurance for in-state students at public institutions in 2018 is $38,119. It gets worse for private schools ($61,533), out-of-state students at public schools ($64,147), and DO

J. M. Dahle (✉)
The White Coat Investor, LLC, Salt Lake City, UT, USA
e-mail: editor@whitecoatinvestor.com

© Springer Nature Switzerland AG 2019
D. Zappetti, J. D. Avery (eds.), *Medical Student Well-Being*,
https://doi.org/10.1007/978-3-030-16558-1_8

students ($51,218 in-state and $54,205 out-of-state, not including health insurance.) To make matters worse, half of the schools are charging more than this. The most expensive school charges over $99,000 per year! But wait, there's more. This doesn't include living expenses, fees for mandatory licensure testing, books, other study materials like question banks, equipment, and residency interviewing-related expenses. The amazing thing is not that the average indebted graduating student reports a total educational debt of $200,000, but that the amount is not higher! For many students, it is. Over 12% report owing over $300,000 in student loans.

Honestly, I am skeptical that even these numbers are accurate. I remember taking this survey myself. It is given before medical school is even over, and respondents typically do not have their financial paperwork in front of them. Many are simply guessing at how much they owe and have not actually added it all up before answering the question. To make matters worse, the debt generally worsens dramatically during residency. At 7% interest with loans in forbearance, $200,000 in debt at medical school graduation has become $281,000 by completion of a 5-year residency. At a median physician income of $300,000, paying that debt off over 10 years will require more than 13% of gross income to be dedicated just to debt payments. Things look even worse for those with above-average debt burdens and below-average income. Consider a medical student who owes $400,000 upon graduation, spends 3 years in pediatrics residency, and then earns $180,000 per year. This doc will need to dedicate 39% of gross income to pay the loans off in the first decade after residency! Depending on tax burden, that is likely over 50% of take-home pay. It is very difficult to save for retirement, pay off other debts, save up a down payment, or save for the college of your own children when more than half of your income is going toward your student loans.

Some medical students have access to substantial financial resources during medical school. Like many highly educated people, they come from a higher socioeconomic class than the general population. In 2017, approximately 23% of medical students come from families in the top 5% by income. 50% of students come from the top income quintile and nearly 80% come from the top two quintiles. These statistics explain why 28% of students graduate from medical school without any student loan debt at all, giving them a significant advantage over their peers.

Medical school is still accessible to those without any financial resources, but attendance will require a lot more sacrifice during the early career. These students will either need to make commitments to an organization like the military or borrow heavily to pay rapidly rising tuition, mandatory fees, and living costs.

Despite these incredible financial stresses, medical students receive little to no training in business, personal finance, investing, or loan management. Typically, any training received is limited to 1 hour of student loan-related counseling given to the class as a whole by someone in the financial aid office with a severe financial conflict of interest.

Is there any doubt that starting a career like this does not promote wellness? Of course not. I have been working at The White Coat Investor for the last 8 years helping doctors develop financial literacy and financial wellness. While the aggregated statistics above look terrible, things are even worse when you meet the individuals struggling under these burdens. The emails I receive describe tears, feelings of shame, sleepless nights, divorce, hopelessness, and vast disappointment. What a dramatic difference from the people that wrote their idealistic admissions essays just a few years earlier! Here's an example of a recent one:

> I know you hear lots of people's financial woes. I almost never read articles that include situations similar to ours, and am beginning to feel that we are way out of the norm. My partner and I both went to one of the most expensive medical schools in California. With tuition and living expenses, our combined debts currently stand at 840K (about 420K each), with interest accruing at about 6.5% for half the amount, and 7.6% for the other half. We are both in residency, Psych and IM.

These sorts of loan burdens require drastic financial solutions. Medical school loans are not Monopoly money, they will have to be paid back eventually, and with after-tax dollars.

In the remainder of this chapter, I aim to provide information and suggestions that will bring hope and control to the chaotic financial lives of young physicians and students. Not every suggestion will be helpful to you, but hopefully there will be at least one pearl you can implement this week to improve your financial life.

Let us begin with the pre-med years. I suspect that most of those reading this book are already in medical school, but in the event that a few readers are not, here are few suggestions.

Pre-med Financial Tips

First, evaluate whether medicine is really the correct career for you. Realize that while medicine is a relatively sure path to a high income, if you put in the time and effort required in the long medical training pipeline into many other fields, you are likely to be even more financially successful. There are many ways to contribute to the world besides medicine, and a fair number of them are easier and pay better. The old saying, "If you can be talked out of medicine, you should be" contains a lot of truth. It takes a firm commitment that this is what you want to do for the rest of your life to get through the decade-long medical training pipeline, much less even half a career in medicine.

Once you have decided that medicine is for you, don't delay. Every year you spend in college, working on a Masters degree, or preparing for the MCAT is a year you are not earning an attending physician salary. In that respect, an unnecessary Master's degree may be an "$800,000 mistake." Now, everything in life isn't about money, but ignorance about the financial ramifications of decisions is often regretted later.

If you are like most medical students and anticipate borrowing to pay for your medical education, do all that you can to leave your undergraduate institution debt-free. While it is very difficult to pay for medical school without borrowing, it is relatively easy to do this at the undergraduate level by careful school selection, calling upon even limited family resources, working during the summers and part-time during the school year, and applying for many scholarships. Starting medical school $50–100,000 in the hole from undergraduate puts you way behind the eight ball and your peers.

One exception to the above involves a rarely used but potentially useful technique. It turns out that undergraduate student loans, unlike their medical school counterparts, have lower interest rates and can be subsidized by the government. If possible, you may wish to consider borrowing some money late in your senior year and then using it to help pay for the first semester of medical school.

If you are a competitive enough applicant that you are accepted to more than one medical school, the classic advice of "Go to the cheapest school you can get into" can be pretty handy. Medical school tuition varies widely, as does the cost of living in the cities where the schools are located. Like with undergraduate institutions, the quality of the education is not necessarily correlated with the cost, and often times is inversely related! Some of the best institutions in any given region of the country are often among the cheapest.

Consider carefully how you will pay for medical school. While most students will take out student loans, a significant portion will instead trade their time for money and make a commitment to an organization such as the military. The classic example here is the military Health Professions Scholarship Program (HPSP), but there are similar programs with the National Guard, the National Health Service Corps (NHSC), Indian Health Services (IHS), and others. MD/PhD programs may also offer living stipends and waived tuition in exchange for your time in the PhD portion of the program.

The HPSP is best thought of not as a scholarship but as a contract. In exchange for paying your tuition, fees, books, and equipment and providing a monthly stipend ($2279.10 for the 2018–2019 year), the military will dictate your life for a few months during medical school, potentially affect your residency selection, and control where you live and work for 4 years as an attending. For many specialties, the military will pay you dramatically less than you would earn as a civilian. You have essentially traded getting the money up front and a few years of control over your life for student loans. Whether that is a good trade or not primarily boils down to your desire to be a military doctor. If this is something you wish to do out of a desire to serve or some unique aspects of military medicine, then you might as well apply for HPSP (or attend the military medical school – Uniformed Services University of the Health Sciences, USUHS.) If being a military physician for at least a few years is not one of your career goals, then you will likely regret signing the contract. Similar reasoning should be used with the other providers of medical school funding.

Medical School Financial Tips

Your primary focus in medical school should be learning how to be a great doctor. It can be a busy time in life, although your workload varies significantly over the 4-year period. Some of the rotations in the third year will be all consuming, as will your preparation for the first step of your licensing exams. However, other periods, particularly the last half of your fourth year, will allow you time to divert some focus toward your finances.

The most important financial consideration in medical school is making sure you actually live like a student. Even if you previously had another career that paid well and allowed you a higher standard of living, you still don't get a pass on math. The fact remains that your income will be very low for 4 years and your expenses will be very high. To make matters worse, a large percentage of your expenses will be fixed expenses, particularly tuition- and school-related fees. You must learn how to live frugally in order to reduce the remaining expenses as much as possible.

It may help you to live frugally when you realize that the effect of compound interest on your relatively high-interest rate loans is to double or even triple the price of everything you buy. That $25 restaurant meal doesn't seem too bad, but you wouldn't pay $75 for it. Same with that $6000 trip to Florida and that $60,000 car. Triple everything in your mind and you'll spend less.

In medical school, everyone expects you to be poor. That will not be the case later on, even though your net worth will actually be even lower. In fact, many of your friends, family, and even patients don't realize that a resident income has far more in common with minimum wage than a typical physician income. But everyone knows you're broke in medical school, so there are no expectations for you to be able to live the high life. Take advantage!

Housing will be a major expense, but can be reduced by living with roommates and getting only what you need. Transportation is also a major expense. However, at many medical schools in major cities, you can avoid owning a car at all. A bicycle is not only inexpensive, but will keep you in great shape. Mr. Money Mustache, a popular finance blogger, has called it a "money-printing fountain of youth." The subway or bus may also meet most or all of your needs. Even if you need a car occasionally, you can use ride-sharing or car-sharing services. If you do buy a car, keep it inexpensive. It won't impress anyone, but reliable transportation can be had for $5–10,000. Keep the costs down, especially if you will be buying it on credit.

Some food is more expensive than other food. Bringing lunch from home is usually much cheaper than visiting the cafeteria each day. There can be a surprising amount of free food available in a medical center. Find out where it is. When you decided to attend medical school, you decided to pass on activities that others your age will be doing during those years. You will have opportunities to go on ski trips, European vacations, and Christmas in Mexico later. For now, you need to learn four words- "I can't afford that." Repeat them until you believe them, because they're true. This can be difficult when you see how other medical students are living and spending. Remember two things that will help you restrain yourself when you see that happening: First, 27% of medical students will graduate debt-free. That's because up to 60% of your class comes from a family in the top income quintile. If you do not, you're in a very different financial situation than they are. Second, the time to pay the piper will come and it takes a significant amount of time and sacrifice, even on an attending physician salary, to pay for the difference between a frugal medical student and a spendthrift medical student.

There are government programs that are designed for poor people. Medical students generally have little income and little assets and so frequently qualify for these assistance programs, particularly if they have children. These programs include subsidized housing, Medicaid, CHIP, and food stamps. Look into these programs, how they work, whether or not you qualify for them, and what you need to do to receive the benefits. I assure you that you will have classmates on these programs, so if you qualify, you should take advantage. The applications do not ask for your potential future income. This is no different than using a tax deduction that you may qualify for. Thanks to our progressive income tax system, if you are like a typical doctor, you will pay far more in taxes over the course of your career than you will ever receive back in benefits from the government, even if the birth of your first child is paid for by Medicaid.

Another little known tactic used by financially savvy medical students is to delay taking out your student loans. There is no requirement that you take out all of the expenses for the entire school year in August. Since medical school loans are no longer subsidized, interest starts accruing from "Day One." So delay "Day One" as long as you can. Since it usually only takes a couple of weeks from application until the money is in your hands, it's okay to only borrow the money as the money is needed. A few medical students have even taken this to an extreme. If they qualify for high enough credit limits, they put their living expenses and even tuition on 0% introductory credit card offers. They roll this debt forward to new cards every 12–15 months as long as they can, only taking out student loans to pay off the cards when the interest rates rise and they can no longer transfer the debt to another low-interest rate card. In this way, the interest that accumulates during medical school can be dramatically reduced. Obviously, it is critical to keep careful track of cards if you go down this route. It doesn't take very many months at typical credit card interest rates to completely eliminate the benefit you're aiming for here.

Medical school is a lot of work. You spend countless hours studying during the first 2 years, and then it gets worse. Many students worry they would not be able to complete their scholastic requirements and hold down any sort of a paying job. However, the intensity of medical school is highly variable. Some classes are easier than others and some rotations are more demanding than others. There may even be large breaks in the program, such as between the first and second year or during the fourth year. Many medical students have incorporated paid work into their lives during these years, balancing school, work, and personal lives just as they did during their undergraduate years. As a fourth year medical student, a number of medical students at my school did pre-surgical history and physicals at a local outpatient surgery center for $20 per hour. In 2002, that was a pretty good wage and really helped with the cost of residency interviews and relocation for residency. Other students were paid research fellows, volunteered as research subjects, or even donated various body fluids for cash during school. The more income you obtain from paid work during school, the less you have to borrow. Just don't forget to prioritize the schooling. You don't want to be penny-wise and pound-foolish and not graduate or not match into your desired specialty because you spent too much time working.

If you are married or otherwise have a partner while in school, this is an ideal time for that person to go out and get a job. Even if their job only covers your living costs and pays nothing toward tuition, it will dramatically reduce your indebtedness. My spouse worked full-time throughout most of my medical school years, including when she went back to school herself for a master's degree. If your spouse is in healthcare, be sure to consider having them work at the university hospital. Many universities offer benefits to the family members of employees, including free or reduced tuition. If your tuition is $60 K per year and you get half off for your spouse working, that's like getting a raise of $30 K per year (or more if the benefit is tax-free.) If your spouse is staying home to care for kids, consider online side hustles. Every little bit counts when the alternative is borrowing at 6–7%.

Some nontraditional medical students enter medical school with cash on hand from their prior work. This money is often best used for school and living costs (i.e., investing in your future earnings ability and saving all that interest). Even if the money is in a retirement account, you can often get it out penalty-free if it is used for education, and given your new low tax bracket, it may also come out completely or nearly tax-free. Another great strategy to consider for those entering medical school with money in a tax-deferred retirement account such as a 401(k) or Individual Retirement Arrangement (IRA) is to do Roth conversions of that money during medical school. Since you have minimal if any income, there may be no tax cost whatsoever to these conversions. Spread out over the 4 years of medical school, even a six-figure sum could be converted to a Roth IRA tax-free.

Medical school is also a great time to begin your financial education, particularly late in the fourth year. The information has a lot more personal meaning and value as you get closer to what for most traditional medical students is their first real paycheck as an intern. Personal finance and investing has its own language and terminology, just like medicine. Just as you need to know the difference between hematopoiesis and gluconeogenesis, you need to know the difference between a 401(k) and a Roth IRA, a marginal and an effective tax rate, and a residual disability rider and a cost of living rider. Your initial financial education should consist of reading three or four high-quality financial books. I recommend one on personal finance, one on investing, one on behavioral finance, and a physician-specific finance book. There are lots of good books in each of these categories (although more bad than good) and more coming out all the time. Consider the following:

- The Only Investment Guide You'll Ever Need by Andrew Tobias
- The Investor's Manifesto by William Bernstein, MD
- How To Think About Money by Jonathan Clements
- The White Coat Investor by James Dahle, MD

Other methods of obtaining your initial financial education include online courses or hiring a fee-only financial advisor to teach you.

Following your initial financial education, you can begin the lifelong process of Continuing Financial Education (CFE.) I recommend you read one good financial book per year and follow a good physician-specific financial blog such as The White Coat Investor. Ideally, by becoming financially educated now, you will hit the ground running as an attending. The secret to financial success as a physician is really all about those first few years out of residency and how much of your new-found high income goes toward building wealth. By maintaining your resident lifestyle while earning as an attending for just 2–5 years, you can rapidly pay off your student loans, save up a down payment on your dream house, and catch up to your college roommates with retirement savings. Aim to have a written financial plan by the time you finish residency so you don't grow into that attending income all at once. I assure you it is far harder to cut back once you have grown into that income than to just grow into it slowly.

Your attending years, unfortunately, probably still feel a long ways off. They sit on the other side of years of sleepless nights and 80-hour work weeks. You will also need a financial plan as a resident, the most important aspect of which will be your student loan management plan. Attending physician student loan management is relatively straightforward, but it can be complicated as a resident. There are a few key principles however.

First, if you have private loans, it is okay to refinance them upon finishing school. They will not be eligible for the government Income Driven Repayment (IDR) or forgiveness programs. At the time of this writing, there are two private companies who will refinance your loans to a lower rate and offer you a very low ($100) monthly payment during residency. Those loans can then be refinanced again, likely at an even lower rate, upon residency completion.

Second, if you have any federal loans that are not direct federal loans, see if you can consolidate them into a direct federal loan. I'm talking primarily about loans taken out before 2010, usually in the FFEL program. Most federal loans taken out since then are already direct federal loans.

Third, there are basically three IDR programs – Income Based Repayment (IBR), Pay As You Earn (PAYE), and Revised Pay As You Earn (RePAYE). All provide low monthly payments based solely on your income and family size, not your interest rate or size of the loan. The payment is calculated by subtracting 150% of the poverty line for your family size and your location from your income to get your "discretionary income." Required payments are 10% (PAYE, RePAYE) to 15% (IBR) of your discretionary income.

The default option for most residents should be RePAYE. The reason why is that RePAYE has one feature the others do not, an interest subsidy. Basically, if your loan generates $1000 per month in interest, and your payment is $200 per month, half of the other $800 will be forgiven. Of course, $400 will be added to the balance of the loan each month, but $400 is better than $800. This effectively reduces your interest rate. If you are a single resident or are married to a non-earner or a low earner, this will almost always be your payment plan of choice for your federal loans. The effective interest rate under RePAYE will likely be less than any rate available through a private loan refinancer. You can further reduce your payments (possibly increasing the RePAYE interest subsidy) by minimizing your income through the use of tax-deferred retirement accounts, although this must be weighed against the marked benefit of using tax-free (Roth) retirement accounts during these low earning years.

If you are married to a moderate to high earner, your ideal direct federal student loan management plan can become very complicated, very quickly. This is a good time to seek out professional advice. RePAYE may still be the right plan, but if there is no interest rate subsidy due to your household income being too high, there are two other options. The first is to simply refinance the loans with a private lender and begin paying them off. This works well if your ultimate plan as an attending is to work in private practice and pay off your loans yourself.

The second option is far more complicated, but works well for those planning to be directly employed by a nonprofit (501(c)3) or government employer after residency. Many of these doctors plan to have their federal direct loans forgiven via the Public Service Loan Forgiveness (PSLF) program. In this program, any remaining eligible direct loans are forgiven tax-free once 120 qualifying monthly payments have been made toward them. Qualifying payments must be made on-time in one of the following programs, IBR, PAYE, RePAYE, or the standard 10-year repayment plan while being directly employed full-time by a 501(c)3 or government employer. Since most residency and fellowship programs are 501(c)3 employer, all of the payments made during residency count toward these 120 payments, even if the payments are tiny. (In fact, payments of $0 count as well!) The strategy here is to get your payments as low as possible during training in order to maximize the amount left to be forgiven after 10 years of payments. This can be done by maximizing contributions to tax-deferred retirement accounts. Some couples even file their taxes Married Filing Separately (MFS) while working toward PSLF. While this does generally increase the taxes due, it can also dramatically lower the required IDR payments and increase the amount left to be forgiven. If you choose to go this route, you will need to use the PAYE program, since RePAYE doesn't provide the same advantage for those filing MFS.

If you are not sure if you will be going for PSLF after residency, it is probably best to hedge your bets and remain in a government IDR program until you are sure. There are also forgiveness programs built into IBR, PAYE, and RePAYE that do not require working full-time for a nonprofit. Unfortunately, in these programs, you have to make payments for 20–25 years instead of 10 and the forgiveness received is fully taxable. Since most doctors will have paid off their loans long before 20 years, these programs should really only be considered by those with a very high student loan debt-to-gross income ratio (>2X). In the event this plan is right for you, you will need to start saving up a side fund for the "tax bomb" that will hit the year the debt is forgiven. It is entirely possible that the eventual tax bill will be larger than the original loan!

Your resident financial plan should also include obtaining disability insurance, and if someone else (such as a spouse or children) depends on your income, term life insurance. Although you may even need these insurance policies as a medical student, it is hard to justify paying for them with borrowed dollars and insurance companies will only sell you a limited amount due to your low income anyway. Thus, most financially savvy doctors buy these critical insurance policies in their first few months of residency. Be sure that any disability insurance policy you buy as a resident includes a specialty-specific own-occupation definition of disability, a partial/residual disability rider, a future purchase option rider, and a cost of living adjustment rider.

One last financial consideration for medical students is to consider the financial ramifications of your residency match list. While the most important aspects of your residency selection should be fit with the residents and attendings in the program and the quality of the education, location matters a great deal too. The variation in residency pay is relatively minor, so I wouldn't put a lot of weight there, but there is no doubt that choosing a residency program in the Midwest is going to leave you a lot more spending money than one in Manhattan or the Bay Area. You may also obtain financial benefit by choosing a program whose location allows you to live with family or where family is available to help with childcare. These financial aspects should be included in the decision process.

Part of wellness is financial wellness and medical students should begin addressing this critical aspect in their education and overall lives early. The freedom that comes with eliminating financial worries will make you a better person, spouse, parent, and physician.

References

1. https://www.aamc.org/data/tuitionandstudentfees/
2. https://www.aamc.org/data/gq/
3. https://www.aacom.org/reports-programs-initiatives/ aacom-reports/entering-and-graduating-class-surveys
4. https://www.med.navy.mil/Accessions/Pages/Pay.aspx
5. https://www.medscape.com/slideshow/2018-compensation-overview-6009667#1
6. https://studentaid.ed.gov/sa/repay-loans/understand/plans/ income-driven
7. https://studentaid.ed.gov/sa/sites/default/files/public-service-employment-certification-form.pdf
8. https://studentaid.ed.gov/sa/sites/default/files/public-service-application-for-forgiveness.pdf

Chapter 9
Beyond Graduation: Next Steps in Wellness

Janna S. Gordon-Elliott

Just imagine: it's mile 26 of a marathon, with 0.2 miles to go. You've been preparing for this for what seems like forever – putting in hours of training, making sacrifices, and preparing a race strategy – in order to perform at your best. You have considered what it will feel like to cross the finish but have also allowed that to come somewhat as a surprise. Training to run 26.2 miles and training to become a doctor are not dissimilar: each, a long haul full of delayed gratification, discomfort, excitement, and hope; and at the end there is a new identity – a marathon finisher, a physician. The medical student's journey does not end at that single finish line. While medical school has been training the student for the next step (i.e., residency and physicianhood), much of the student's focus has been on graduation, a residency position, and preparing to be ready to competently perform on day one of internship. That finish line, however, is just the next step of a lengthy and demanding journey that will test even the hardiest contenders.

J. S. Gordon-Elliott (✉)
New York Presbyterian Hospital/Weill Cornell Medical College,
New York, NY, USA
e-mail: jsg2005@med.cornell.edu

© Springer Nature Switzerland AG 2019   171
D. Zappetti, J. D. Avery (eds.), *Medical Student Well-Being*,
https://doi.org/10.1007/978-3-030-16558-1_9

While those starting medical school do not demonstrate elevated prevalence of psychiatric illness, this changes as they progress through training and their careers, with rising risk for emotional distress, substance use, and mental health disorders. Rates of depression and burnout are higher among physicians than for age-matched controls, and suicide rates are nearly 1.5 and more than 2 times population averages for men and women physicians, respectively [12]. Impaired well-being among physicians may negatively impact empathy, work satisfaction, and quality of patient care [14]. Arguably, attending to one's well-being is an essential component of physician professionalism and something that the medical student should be considering in anticipation of residency and beyond [4].

As the student looks ahead to graduation, that initial goal is now in clear sight, but what lies beyond it may be less perceptible. Having knowledge of the personal and professional challenges ahead and considering how they can be endured – and even welcomed – will benefit the emerging physician. Preparing for lifelong wellness will involve anticipating the difficulties that may arise during residency and later stages of one's career, and developing the resilience and skills to adapt and flourish.

Living with Stress

The Stress Response

While the word stress carries a negative connotation for many, it is important to consider the purpose, course, and impact of stress. The stress response is a normal function that is generated in order to address a stimulus that requires attention or action. Necessary for survival, the *acute stress response* involves an increase in sympathetic tone, enhanced cognitive focus, and redirection of our resources to respond to a salient experience – e.g., running from a lion, studying for a major exam. It lasts for a matter of minutes to hours. Our physiologic and mental response to acute stress may be uncomfortable (e.g., pounding heart rate, feeling frightened), or positively activating (e.g., feeling "on", energized, or excited). A panic attack is an example of a malfunctioning of the acute stress response: activation of the autonomic nervous system in response to a thought or other stimulus that is not, in fact, a major threat. In many cases, however, the acute stress response does not need to be feared or considered unsafe. Facing high-priority situations with a degree of urgency or necessity helps us to learn, grow, and potentially become stronger. Brief stress, for example, can assist with memory consolidation and accuracy of cognitive performance [5, 11]. Without intermittent challenges, we would likely learn less, develop fewer new skills, and perhaps even feel unstimulated. A muscle strengthens from progressive overload – increasing the intensity of the load on the muscle – to the limit of or just beyond the muscle's capacity and then allowing for a period of rest during which the muscle adapts to that new load. Common daily stressors serve the same purpose for our emotional and cognitive resilience, as long as a few criteria are met: that we – like the muscle – are not tested too far beyond our limits, have the durability to manage the progressive load, and are given adequate time for recovery in between these challenges.

Problems can arise in response to stress if those criteria are consistently not met, or if the individual being stressed has particular vulnerabilities such as a mental health condition, limited coping skills in response to stress, or excessive burden of additive stress, which threaten that person's ability to manage the stress of the new stimulus. Acute challenges that feel unfamiliar and without context, significantly beyond our capacities or control, or lacking in clarity or predictability, can be particularly problematic for most; such situations may – rather than stimulating growth – lead to maladaptive responses (such as negative thoughts and emotions) and vulnerability. When a stressor becomes chronic, or when there is a cumulative burden of many stressors, there is insufficient recovery. In this *chronic stress response*, continuous activation of the stress system negatively impacts health in a variety of systems, from immunity, to cardiovascular, to cognitive and emotional. Learning and memory are impaired in chronic stress. Learned helplessness, anger, depression, anxiety, substance use, reduced job performance, and relationship difficulties are all possible outcomes over time.

Burnout

Burnout is a specific consequence of chronic stress that is worth further mention. An individual may develop burnout in the context of an uninterrupted stress that is perceived as emotionally taxing, largely outside of one's control, and subject to high external demands. Often associated with an occupation, burnout presents with a range of mental and physical symptoms, and has been defined by the core features of emotional exhaustion, depersonalization, and reduction in one's sense of personal accomplishment [7]. "I have nothing left to give," or "I'm spent" may be how the experience is described. Empathy and generosity wane or feel burdensome; cynicism grows. Work-related pleasure and motivation decline.

Individual and organization/system level factors that increase susceptibility to burnout are known as *drivers* of burnout. In the healthcare field, system-based drivers include, though are not limited to, high workload and clerical demands, limited administrative support, conflicts between work and nonwork priorities, and organizational structures that restrain professional autonomy. Individual drivers include life stressors such as inadequate or conflictual social support, and financial debt. On the individual level, demographic and personality-related features that may also be associated with development of burnout include being female gender, or of nonminority status, and tendencies toward excessive worry or self-critical thinking. Exposure to supervisors with burnout may impact the well-being, and burnout risk, of trainees [3, 9, 15].

The implications of burnout are significant, including increasing risk for poor physical health, depression, substance use, and suicidal ideation; interpersonal withdrawal or conflict; less optimal patient care, unprofessional behavior, and an increased rate of medical errors; early departure from direct patient care or from medicine, entirely; and financial losses and reduced access to care across the broader healthcare system [16].

Physicians have high rates of burnout. This may not come as a surprise: personal traits and experiences that are common in medicine (such as exacting standards for oneself, high degrees of conscientiousness, years of delay of gratification, and financial debt), combined with aspects of the medical culture and system (e.g., the intense nature of working with sickness and death, the needs of patients and families, the rising complexity and constraints of the healthcare system, and the prioritization of serving others, often at the expense of one's own needs), can strain even the most resilient individuals and may lead to burnout if the right personal and organizational efforts are not in place. Indeed, physicians consistently have higher rates of burnout than age-matched peers. Ostensibly, this is not because they are already more emotionally vulnerable at baseline. At the start of training, medical students do not have higher rates of burnout or mental health issues than peers pursuing other rigorous professions. By the end of medical school, up to 50% of students may have features, or the full syndrome, of burnout, and this appears to rise over residency [3]. Rates of burnout, distress, and dissatisfaction remain high as physicians progress through early and mid-career. Once thought to be a consequence of years of work, burnout, and lower-grade emotional effects of chronic work stress can have their origins early in training, and must be actively addressed. Notably – with implications on prevention and management – current research indicates that organizational/system level drivers are more influential in the development of burnout than are the individual-based factors, including personality traits, behaviors, and attitudes.

The Transitions to, Through, and Beyond Residency

The student approaching residency looks ahead to a future marked by many stressors, acute and chronic, over a career and a lifetime (Table 9.1). Some stressors can be adjusted,

TABLE 9.1 Events and stressors relevant to work and life

Work-related factors	Personal factors
Residency and fellowship	*Timeline may vary among individuals*
• Adjusting from *student* to *employed trainee*	• Housing and location: e.g., uprooting to a new location, finding housing, paying rent, or buying a home
• Adapting to the responsibility of the MD role, making critical decisions	
• Adjusting to new forms of feedback	• Adapting to new communities: e.g., colleagues, other social contacts
• Gaining mastery in the clinical work	
• Supervising junior trainees	• Relationships: e.g., friends, partner, marriage, divorce
• Acculturation to specialty identity	• Family: e.g., planning for and raising children; caring for aging parent; illness in family, pets
• Considering next steps	
Post-training career	• Health: e.g., establishing personal health care (health insurance, primary care provider, dentist, etc.); developing and adjusting self-care habits to fit around work schedules
• Adjusting from *trainee* to *employee*	
• Adapting to the role and responsibilities of being the attending	
• Supervising residents and fellows	• Financial: e.g., housing, debt, planning for retirement
• Learning about the system, e.g., reporting and oversight hierarchy, administrative aspects of medicine, teaching, and academic responsibilities	
• Adjusting to a longer, less linear, less punctuated timeline for the future	

some tolerated; some will spur growth, and some will prompt problematic reactions. Anticipating many of these potential stressors and planning in advance for ways to manage them can enhance the lifelong wellness of the developing physician, personally and professionally.

Residency and Fellowship

Post-graduate medical training is a time of substantial professional and personal adjustment, high stress, and notable mental health burdens. Studies have consistently found lower scores of well-being in residents compared to their nonphysician peers [10]. Rates of depressive symptoms are significantly higher than population averages [8]. In a 2018 Medscape survey of 1900 residents from a wide range of specialties, nearly one-half of respondents reported feeling depressed some or all of the time, ten percent reported having had thoughts of suicide, and more than two-thirds of those responding reported "sometimes" or "always/most of the time" having doubts about being a "good physician" [6].

While every incoming resident's experience will be unique, there are characteristic stressors that will manifest in some way for most during the transition to post-graduate training. The work, itself, will pose many new challenges. While many of the tasks will feel familiar, the tone of the work may seem quite different. The new responsibility of being the doctor – the one who puts in orders, who is called with critical laboratory values, and who is paged with emergencies – can be thrilling, motivating, and daunting. Increasing competence will bring confidence; the new pressures may also bring self-doubt. Worries about making mistakes may prompt new tendencies to check and recheck orders, or revisit decisions after the fact. On the one hand, these may be healthy signs of conscientiousness, important when it comes to a job where lives hang in the balance; on the other hand, when such behaviors become more extreme, they can lead to lack of rest, troubling anxiety, and significant emotional distress.

Additionally, the new resident will be taking on a new role as a supervisor to others – initially supervising students and, over time, junior residents. Teaching others can be the most effective route to mastery, though it can also be challenging, such as when the resident is learning to balance teaching with completing tasks, or when feeling uneasy or insecure embodying the authority of the supervisor role. Similarly, the resident will be adjusting to a new relationship with supervisors. Compared to the attending-student relationship, the attending-resident relationship will operate differently. The attending may engage more directly with the resident, have higher expectations of the resident, be more dependent on the resident for patient care, and be less tolerant of errors or gaps in knowledge. This new collaboration can be exciting and challenging. There may be a sense of newfound confidence in being the one who enacts the plan the attending decides on, and even devising the plan that the attending agrees with; there might also be worry about making mistakes, or of being judged harshly. The feedback process, in addition, may be new. Whereas the student may have been accustomed to formal feedback given at the midpoint or end of a rotation, the resident may not have as clear an idea of how or when feedback will be given, or may experience getting limited or intermittent feedback, or only receiving feedback after an adverse outcome, in which case the content and tone may be primarily critical.

The transition to post-graduate training involves adjustments and challenges in the personal sphere. Graduation from medical school often comes at a time of, or brings with it, other significant life changes. Many residents are moving to a new city or area of the country, sometimes for a first-choice program, and sometimes after a disappointing match. They might be moving away from loved ones, to a place where they have few roots or connections, and this may be frightening, or even liberating. For those moving back to a familiar area for the first time since college or childhood, there may be positive emotions as well as new work-family conflicts to maneuver. The resident may be rushing to find an apartment to live in; this might be the first experience renting an apartment not provided by student housing services, or the first time covering rent independently with one's salary. Not uncommonly, transitions in committed relationships overlap with beginning of residency – some new residents are cohabiting with their partners for the first time, some have just married. Similarly, the start of residency may follow the termination of relationships, either because of moving for the match or other life factors. From a community point of view, friendships may change during this adjustment to residency. Some residents are in new locations, having to make new friends, and feeling separation from old friends; for others, pressures related to becoming a resident, anticipating long hours or few off-days, may have led to gradual withdrawal from, or changes in, some friendships. Adjusting to one's new residency class can be satisfying, while in some situations can bring anxiety and feelings of insecurity. Additional personal changes at various points in training will test the resident's well-being, positively, and otherwise. Relationship difficulties, starting a family and raising children, and health issues – both personal and those of loved ones – will all happen without much respect for the resident's responsibilities or ideal "timeline."

Personal care is another element of life which will need conscious attention during this transition and beyond. Whether the resident is in a new location or not, there will likely be need to establish a new primary care provider – either due to new insurance or loss of access to the student health physician. The same may apply to one's mental health treatment, where applicable. This may also be the first time the individual is managing health insurance alone, perhaps having been on a parent's plan until this point or because health insurance was managed by school. Due to changes in work schedule, lifestyle, or other responsibilities or choices, the resident may also have to develop a new personal care routine, from exercise, to eating, to sleep.

Identity, both personal and professional, will be challenged during this transition to and through post-graduate training. First is the shift to the identity of the resident physician.

There may be tension in adjusting to this new role. The individual is now officially a physician and is now employed as a worker; and yet while not still a student, still a trainee. As an employee, perhaps the first significant job as adult, there will be expectations to provide service and to meet compliance standards. At the same time, the resident is also an apprentice, receiving education on the job. The demands to work and to learn may conflict at times, and even lead to some degree of role confusion. In addition, in this new role, performance and capability is no longer measured by a grade, but now by more of a complex extrapolation of many points of data, including patient outcomes, feedback received from attendings, students, nurses, and program directors, and an imprecise sense of "how I think I'm doing."

As training progresses, the resident acculturates to the identity of the chosen specialty. This process may provide the resident with an enhanced sense of belonging and a confirmation of having made the "right choice"; whereas for some, it may provoke doubts about being a good "fit" within that specialty, or even within the profession of medicine. The mid- to late phases of residency will also force decisions about the next step – what to do after residency. This may mean having to prepare for another match for a desired fellowship, with the associated stressors related to compiling an application, interviewing, and prioritizing programs. As training nears its end, the search for the first post-training job will begin. New challenges may include facing insecurities about clinical independence, choosing among an array of options without a match system to make the final decision, and knowing one's "worth" and engaging in negotiations with potential employers. The "impostor syndrome," in which the individual doubts personal accomplishments and experiences an internalized sense of being a "fraud" who is "about to be found out" – one that may rear its head at many points during medical training – may feel particularly acute at this point.

This phase may also provoke questions about what the next step should be. Perhaps for the first time – after 20 years of school, and several years of professional training – there may not be a clearly visualized path ahead. This can be exciting, but also unnerving. The decision is no longer limited to "which program" or "which subspecialty," but involves broader questions such as "what kind of setting do I want to practice in?", "how do I want to practice?", and "what will feel most satisfying to me?" This may be a period when the resident first really grapples with questions of personal priorities and choices, in contrast to following a defined trajectory and the instructions of others. There may be consideration of life-work balance. Depending on individual needs, there may be decisions about full- vs. part-time work, choices that raise anxieties about time with family and financial compensation. This phase may stimulate even deeper self-reflection about how medicine has changed the person – for good and for bad. With this may come meaningful insight and personal satisfaction, or disillusionment, resentment, and anxiety.

Transitions Beyond Training

Many of the stressors faced by the medical student and post-graduate trainee will remain relevant to the physician throughout a career. Certain challenges may specifically arise during the transition from trainee to junior attending and over subsequent career development. Just as during the transition to residency, the new attending will experience familiar work through a new perspective. Now the "final word" on medical decisions, and the "attending of record," this authority may be experienced as freeing and frightening. New reporting structures and administrative responsibilities that were not present during training will become apparent. As time goes on, the physician may have to learn to split time between clinical work and other academic and departmental responsibilities. There will be encouragement and even pressure to take on additional roles and tasks; seizing worthwhile opportunities, while knowing when and how to say "no," will be a challenging balancing act that might test the physician's sense of identity and assumed priorities.

As mid-career approaches, the physician may start to question the future again. While the relative stability of the physician's job, compared to the constant upheavals of training, may allow for more security and a sense of evolving competency, it may also lead to feelings of monotony – realizations that, unlike residency, this could be "forever." As did the search for the first job after training, this period may prompt reflection about priorities, including the kind of setting and type of demands the individual feels will be optimal. As part of this process, doubts about career and life aspirations may arise, and for some there may even be consideration of alternate careers outside of clinical medicine.

The various life stressors that were applicable to the resident experience may occur at any point during the physician's career. There may be relocations to new institutions or new locations, sometimes because of personal choice and sometimes not. There may be marriages, divorces, health matters, child-rearing, and new responsibilities caring for aging and ailing parents that the physician will be invested in, challenged by, and fulfilled by, along the way.

Interventions

Many of the transition periods and common stressors so far described, and many others, will test the developing physician in all of the same ways medical school did and with the same potential implications. Stress that exceeds one's usual coping mechanisms and resilience can impair physical and mental health, performance at work, relationship functioning and satisfaction, and personal fulfillment. The physician will be vulnerable to emotional distress, maladaptive behaviors, burnout, depression, substance use, and suicidality; there may be recrudescence of prior mental health issues. Barriers to care, including stigma associated with mental health treatment, may prevent or limit the effectiveness of treatment. Strain on well-being has a cumulative effect; the student who enters residency already depleted may be more susceptible to further mental health difficulties during residency. While some periods of stress and increased vulnerability can be anticipated, the content or timing of each stressor may not always be able to be predicted. What can be predicted, however, is that these vulnerable points *will* happen. And with a bit of attention, forethought, and self-awareness, the emerging physician can be prepared for many of them.

What are ways for physicians and the systems that they work within to build strength and resilience to adapt to stress – and not only endure, but flourish? Much can be learned from the growing literature on burnout. Strategies for preventing and managing burnout are categorized as organization- and individual-based. The organization-based intervention of duty-hours restrictions for post-graduate trainees has been associated with reduction of burnout. Other system-based interventions to promote well-being include creative approaches to enhance flexibility in work schedule and coverage to address work-home conflicts, institutional efforts to improve physician workflow and autonomy, and development of wellness programs with top-down institutional support. Approaches that focus on the individual include involvement in wellness-enhancing activities, such as mindfulness practices, healthy lifestyle practices, and meaningful social engagement [2, 3, 15, 16]. Factors associated with positive wellness in residents include autonomy in one's work, a sense of increasing competence, and strong connections with others [10].

These and other strategies may be useful for minimizing burnout, enhancing resilience to stress, and optimizing wellness; a combination of efforts may be synergistic (Fig. 9.1). Healthcare systems can invest in the well-being of their physicians through establishment of wellness programs – coordinated efforts which may include streamlined access to healthcare and health-promoting activities and initiatives that enhance the work experience and autonomy of physicians (such as reducing redundancy in required tasks and documentation, and improving administrative support). Stanford University has developed a premiere wellness program, WellMD, with an

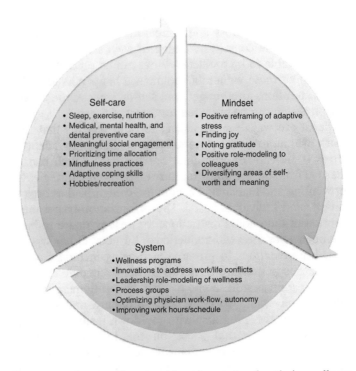

Self-care
- Sleep, exercise, nutrition
- Medical, mental health, and dental preventive care
- Meaningful social engagement
- Prioritizing time allocation
- Mindfulness practices
- Adaptive coping skills
- Hobbies/recreation

Mindset
- Positive reframing of adaptive stress
- Finding joy
- Noting gratitude
- Positive role-modeling to colleagues
- Diversifying areas of self-worth and meaning

System
- Wellness programs
- Innovations to address work/life conflicts
- Leadership role-modeling of wellness
- Process groups
- Optimizing physician work-flow, autonomy
- Improving work hours/schedule

FIGURE. 9.1 Interventions to address burnout and optimize wellness

open-access informative website [13]. A culture of wellness can be encouraged through thoughtful role modeling by leadership. Peer-process groups can be sponsored by the institution to provide opportunities for physicians to explore shared challenges, which may help to validate and normalize their experiences and promote active problem-solving and a sense of community. Individuals can further develop personal wellness by attending to their self-care needs, including physical and emotional health, and prioritizing how they use their time (e.g., allocation of professional efforts, and protection of time and energy for life outside of work).

Conscious adjustment of one's mindset and perspective can be a powerful tool for growing and sustaining wellness over a lifetime. Identifying various sources of meaning, self-worth, and satisfaction in one's life (e.g., viewing onself as a capable physician, a caring parent, and a talented piano player) can help protect one's general sense of competence and self-esteem during difficult times that test one of these areas in particular. Investing oneself in meaningful relationships and nonwork-related activities can buffer against chronic work stress. Seeking out joy in the daily routines of work, such as a connection made with a patient, a helpful lesson taught to a supervisee, or a joke shared with a staff member, may uplift mood and reduce pessimism and demoralization. In its common program requirements, the Accreditation Council for Graduate Medical Education (ACGME) cites *joy* as component of the learning environment for post-graduate trainees [1]. Modeling one's attention to wellness (e.g., by talking openly about seeking mental health support, by demonstrating one's engagement in meaningful activities outside of work, or by discussing the fulfillment one gets from work) among peers, trainees, and other colleagues can have the effect of promoting positive change in others and in the work environment; this can have an enduring impact on one's community and reinforce one's own feelings of gratitude, resilience, and well-being.

Wellness is a state that is not achieved, but an ongoing process requiring continuous effort and intention. To be resilient is to be flexible in response to internal and external pressures and stressors. Filling our wellness reserves during times of plenty – for example, by getting a few extra minutes of sleep, spending quality time with loved ones, or consciously acknowledging gratitude – can help protect us from total depletion during the lean times. Becoming aware of areas of personal weakness and learning to address those weak spots and anticipate stressors that add further vulnerability are important developmental tasks. And while wellness remains a goal, it is not an absolute antidote. Psychiatric issues warrant assessment and treatment and may threaten well-being for even the most wellness-conscientious physician; hence, the inclusion of psychiatric treatment, when appropriate, as a principle of wellness. Similarly, it is important to recognize when difficulties an individual is facing at work are related to an objectively inappropriate or unacceptable situation, and not a vulnerability or deficit that can be repaired with more attention to personal wellness efforts. While wellness practices are not inherently harmful, over-emphasis of wellness as the individual's responsibility, or the remedy for all difficulties, may have unintended negative consequence, such as demoralization, helplessness, lack of institutional accountability, or inadequately treated mental or physical health issues.

Conclusions

The student approaching graduation has accomplished an impressive task; there is much to be proud of, and much strength that can be taken from having arrived at this point. Remaining resilient for what lies ahead will involve coming up with a strategy that takes into account the long view – knowing one's strengths and weaknesses, and, to the extent that particular challenges can be anticipated, knowing when to surge and when to pace more cautiously. Attending to wellness will remain of fundamental importance to the emerging physician, and a professional responsibility. The process will involve monitoring one's emotional and behavioral needs; finding ways, individually and within the system, to manage chronic stress and optimize well-being; and building resilience to protect against the depleting effects of the major stressors that are bound to emerge. Without conscious attention to this task, the numerous challenges the physician will face – small and large, acute and chronic – may take a toll that will be difficult for the individual to surmount, whereas active efforts to promote well-being will increase the likelihood of a successful and satisfying lifelong experience for the physician.

References

1. Accreditation Council for Graduate Medical Education. ACGME program requirements (residency). 2018. https://www.acgme.org/Portals/0/PFAssets/ProgramRequirements/CPRResidency2019.pdf. Accessed 27 Nov 2018.

2. Busireddy KR, Miller JA, Ellison K, Ren V, Qayyum R, Panda M. Efficacy of interventions to reduce resident physician burnout: a systematic review. J Grad Med Educ. 2017;9:294–301.

3. Dyrbye L, Shanafelt T. A narrative review on burnout experienced by medical students and residents. Med Educ. 2016;50:132–49.

4. Dyrbye LN, Harper W, Moutier C, Duming SJ, Power DV, Massie FS, Eacker A, Thomas MR, Satele D, Sloan JA, Shanafelt TD. A multi-institutional study exploring the impact of positive mental health on medical professionalism in an era of high burnout. Acad Med. 2012;87:1024–31.

5. Kohn N, Hermans EJ, Fernandez G. Cognitive benefit and cost of acute stress is differentially modulated by individual brain state. Soc Cogn Affect Neurosci. 2017;12:1179–87.

6. Levy S. Residency lifestyle & happiness report 2018 (medscape). https://www.medscape.com/slideshow/2018-residents-lifestyle-report-6010110. Accessed 28 Nov 2018.

7. Maslach C, Jackson SE, Leiter MP. Maslach burnout inventory manual. 3rd ed. Palo Alto: Consulting Psychologists Press; 1996.

8. Mata DA, Ramos MA, Bansal N, Khan R, Guille DAE, Sen S. Prevalence of depression and depressive symptoms among resident physicians: a systematic review and meta-analysis. JAMA. 2015;314:2373–83.

9. Patel RS, Bachu R, Adikey A, Malik M, Shah M. Factors related to physician burnout and its consequences: a review. Behav Sci. 2018;8:98.

10. Raj KS. Well-being in residency: a systematic review. J Grad Med Educ. 2016;8:674–84.

11. Sandi C. Stress and cognition. Wiley Interdiscip Rev Cogn Sci. 2013;4:245–61.

12. Schernhammer ES, Colditz GA. Suicide rates among physicians: a quantitative and gender assessment (meta-analysis). Am J Psychiatry. 2004;161:2295–302.

13. Stanford University WellMD. https://wellmd.stanford.edu. Accessed 28 Nov 2018.

14. Wallace JE, Lemaire JB, Ghali WA. Physician wellness: a missing quality indicator. Lancet. 2009;374:1714–21.

15. West CP, Dyrbye LN, Erwin PJ, Shanafelt TD. Interventions to prevent and reduce physician burnout: a systematic review and meta-analysis. Lancet. 2016;388:2272–81.

16. West CP, Dyrbye LN, Shanafelt TD. Physician burnout: contributors, consequences and solutions. J Intern Med. 2018;283:516–29.

Index

Printed in the United States
By Bookmasters